EDIBLE FLOWERS OF THE WORLD

Sébastien Mallet

EDIBLE FLOWERS IN THE WORLD

The 40 edible flowers that heal, virtues of flowers to improve your health

Copyright © 2023 - Avenet Edition

All rights reserved. No part of this book may be reproduced, stored in a retrieval system or transmitted in any form or by any means, electronic, mechanical, photocopying, recording or otherwise, without the prior written permission of the publisher, except in the case of brief quotations incorporated in reviews or newspaper articles.

Disclaimer of liability

Dear Readers, the information presented in this book is intended for educational and informational purposes only. Every effort has been made to ensure the accuracy of this information, its reliability and its verified sources.

The information herein is not intended to be a substitute for professional advice, and the author declines all responsibility for any misinterpretation of this information.

Contents

Introduction	9
Part I: European and Mediterranean edible flowers	17
THE VIOLET	18
NASTURTIUM	22
THE BORAGE	26
THE LAVENDER	30
MARIGOLD	34
THE ROSE	38
LE CORNFLOWER	42
DAISY	46
DAYLILY	50
ZUCCHINI FLOWERS	54
THE PANSY	58
THE LINDEN TREE	62
THE MONARDE	66
Part II: Tropical and Exotic Edible Flowers	71
HIBISCUS	72
JASMINE	76
TAGETE	80
THE ORCHID	84

WATER LILIES	*88*
THE BEGONIA	*92*
BANANA FLOWER	*96*
THE CHRYSANTHEMUM	*100*
THE COCONUT FLOWER	*104*
PLUMBAGO	*108*
THE PASSIFLORA	*112*
THE TUBERUSE	*116*
YLANG-YLANG	*120*
Part III: Wild North American Edible Flowers	**125**
LION'S-TOOTH	*126*
MEADOW SAGE	*130*
RED CLOVER	*134*
DANDELION	*138*
MALLOW	*142*
MYOSOTIS	*146*
FIREWEED	*150*
MARSHMALLOW	*154*
ST. JOHN'S WORT	*158*
OXEYE DAISY	*162*
YARROW	*166*
LILY	*170*

GROUND IVY	*174*
MEADOWSWEET	*178*
Conclusion	**183**

INTRODUCTION

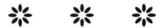

Introducing Edible Flowers

For centuries, flowers have seduced us with their beauty, fragrance and ability to symbolize emotions. They are an integral part of cultures the world over, whether to mark important events, express feelings or simply add a touch of aestheticism to our spaces. But beyond their ornamental role, some flowers also hold unique flavors and health-giving properties, making them valuable components in our diet and well-being.

The notion of an edible flower is part of an ancient tradition. In some civilizations, flowers were used as offerings to the gods, while others consumed them for their nutritional or medicinal qualities. Today, with growing interest in healthy, varied and natural foods, edible flowers are enjoying a veritable renaissance.

Over time, each region of the world has developed a unique relationship with edible flowers, incorporating them into its customs, culinary traditions and remedies. In Europe, for example, violets were appreciated for their delicate taste and used in confectionery. In tropical regions, hibiscus, with its bright red hue and tangy taste, has become a staple of refreshing drinks. Native North American cultures, meanwhile, have drawn on the richness of their local flora to incorporate flowers such as dandelion into their diets and medicinal treatments.

Using flowers in cooking is not just a quest for new flavors. It's also a complete sensory exploration. Their vivid colors can transform an ordinary dish into a work of art, while their textures and aromas add an extra dimension to the culinary experience. What's more, many of these flowers are packed with antioxidants, vitamins and minerals, offering significant nutritional benefits.

But why have flowers been eclipsed from our modern plates for so long? There are many reasons. The standardization of agriculture, changing tastes and a preference for more "conventional" foods have all contributed to reducing the diversity of what we eat. Fortunately, with the rise of innovative culinary movements and the rediscovery of traditional flavors, edible flowers are finding their way back into the kitchens of chefs and food lovers the world over.

Immerse yourself in the world of edible flowers, and you'll realize that nature abounds in treasures that are often unsuspected. It's an invitation to rediscover, through the prism of gastronomy and well-being, the richness and diversity of our environment. An invitation to see nature not only as a visual spectacle, but also as a priceless source of gustatory pleasure.

Importance and Use in Cooking and Medicine

Edible flowers are not simply aesthetic assets or gustatory curiosities; they embody a harmonious marriage between cooking and medicine, two fields in which man has always sought to get the best out of nature.

In the kitchen: Since the dawn of time, gastronomy has been a window on the culture, history and traditions of a society. Integrating flowers into our dishes is much more than a fantasy: it's an art. Their variety of tastes, textures and colors gives chefs the opportunity to reinvent classic dishes or create new culinary experiences. Think of the sweetness of a rose infused into a syrup, or the radiance of a nasturtium adorning a summer salad. These transformative elements make edible flowers a prized ingredient for innovative cooks.

But it's not just in great kitchens that flowers play their part. Many households around the world have been incorporating flowers into their traditional recipes for centuries, from ajowan-scented chapatis to refreshing hibiscus drinks.

In medicine: If we look beyond their culinary appeal, many flowers also have recognized medicinal virtues. Long before the advent of modern medicine, ancient civilizations had discovered the curative properties of certain flowers. Chamomile, for example, has been praised since antiquity for its soothing and anti-inflammatory effects. Similarly, marigold flower is traditionally used for its healing properties.

These ancestral practices, based on observation and experience, paved the way for modern scientific research. Today, many active ingredients extracted from flowers are at the heart of natural medicines and treatments. They are used for everything from skin care to cough remedies, as a testament to nature's healing power.

The interconnection between cooking and medicine through edible flowers perfectly illustrates the notion of "food as medicine". It reminds us that what we eat can not only satisfy our taste buds, but also nourish our bodies and support our well-being.

Far from being mere ornaments, edible flowers are multifunctional pillars that enrich our culinary and medicinal heritage. They encourage us to rethink the way we perceive and use the natural gifts that surround us.

Safety Tips and Precautions

The beauty and richness of edible flowers, though seductive, call for a cautious approach. Incorporating these treasures of nature into our food and medicine must be done with knowledge and discernment. Here are a few essential tips to keep in mind:

1. **Precise identification:** Not all flowers are edible. Before consuming or using a flower, be sure of its exact identity. Mistaken identification can have serious consequences, as some flowers can be toxic.

2. **Provenance:** When buying edible flowers, make sure they have not been treated with pesticides or other chemicals. Choose organic flowers or those specifically labelled as edible.

3. **Moderate consumption:** Even if a flower is edible, this doesn't mean it can be eaten in large quantities. Always start with a small amount to check for allergic reactions or sensitivities.

4. **Medicinal use:** If you wish to use flowers for their medicinal properties, consult a qualified health professional or herbalist. Herbal medicine is powerful and should be approached with respect and caution.

5. **Preserving nature:** When picking flowers in the wild, do so responsibly. Never pick all the flowers on a given plant or in a given area, so as not to disturb the local ecosystem.

6. **Storage:** Edible flowers are delicate. Keep them refrigerated in an airtight container or plastic bag with a sheet of paper towel to preserve their freshness.

7. **Cleaning:** Before eating flowers, it's essential to wash them gently under a trickle of cold water to remove any residue or insects.

8. **Knowing the edible parts:** Not all parts of an edible flower are suitable for consumption. Sometimes only the petals are edible, while other parts may be bitter or less digestible.

Each flower, with its unique color, fragrance and properties, brings a special touch to our table and first-aid kit. However, as with everything, it's essential to approach it with respect, knowledge and caution. By taking these precautions, you can fully enjoy the joys and benefits of edible flowers.

Let's discover the 40 edible flowers together!

Your opinion counts!

Once you've finished this book, share your review on Amazon.

Your feedback will be useful for future readers.

I look forward to seeing how this book has impacted you.

Thank you in advance for your contribution, and happy reading!

PART I: EUROPEAN AND MEDITERRANEAN EDIBLE FLOWERS

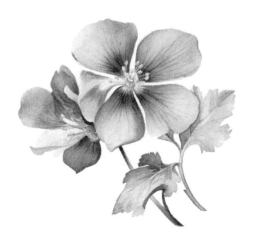

THE VIOLET
(VIOLA)

THE FRAGRANT SWEETNESS OF SPRING

Let's begin our exploration of edible flowers with the violet, a symbol of sweetness and delicacy, much appreciated for its fragrant notes and multiple benefits.

The violet, a small, delicate flower with usually purple petals, has been known since antiquity for its medicinal qualities and its use in cooking. This flower of the Violaceae family is widespread in temperate regions of the northern hemisphere. As far back as medieval times, violets were cultivated in monastic gardens for their purifying and calming properties. The ancient Greeks also used it to make aromatized wines, and it was an essential component of traditional pharmacopoeia. From ancient Rome to the Renaissance, it was prized as much for its delicate aromas as for its medicinal attributes. Violet is said to have expectorant, anti-inflammatory and calming properties.

In the kitchen

Violet is a culinary treasure that brings a delicate fragrance and vibrant color to a variety of preparations. It blends wonderfully into **salads**, adding a **fresh, floral note**. Crystallized petals are a sweet delight and a magnificent decoration for pastries and cakes. **Rich in vitamins A and C**, it adds not only color and flavor, but also **nutritional value**. Its young, tender leaves can be used as a leafy vegetable, adding a pleasant texture and mild flavor to dishes.

In modern culinary art, violets have found their way into **syrups**, liqueurs and even jellies, offering a distinctive taste and bewitching aroma. What's more, its essential oil is often used to **flavor sweets** and desserts, creating a unique gastronomic experience. Not only is violet a feast for the eyes, it also enhances the **taste palette** with its delicate, fragrant presence. Chefs the world over praise its ability to enrich and sublimate even the simplest dishes, adding an elegant floral touch and a certain sophistication.

This little floral treasure offers a wonderful opportunity to explore new flavors and reinvent your favorite recipes with a **fragrant spring note that** will delight every palate.

HEALING WITH VIOLETS

- For **headaches,** infuse a teaspoon of violet flowers in a cup of boiling water for 10 minutes. Strain and drink twice a day.

- For **skin problems**, apply a compress of infused violet flowers directly to the affected area.

- If you suffer from a **cough** or **sore throat**, make an herbal tea with a handful of violet flowers and honey. Drink three times a day.

- To soothe **burns and inflammation,** make a paste of crushed violet flowers and apply to the affected area.

- For **constipation,** take a teaspoon of dried violet flowers with a cup of water, leave to infuse for 15 minutes and drink this infusion in the morning on an empty stomach.

- If you suffer from **insomnia,** use violet flowers as an infusion before bedtime to benefit from its relaxing, soothing properties.

- For **minor cuts and wounds**, apply violet juice directly for its antiseptic and healing properties.

VIOLETS IN THE KITCHEN

Spring Salad with Violet

INGREDIENTS: A few young lettuce leaves, a handful of violet flowers, 1 avocado, 1 cucumber, a few cherry tomatoes, extra virgin olive oil, balsamic vinegar, salt and pepper.

1. Wash and spin-dry the lettuce leaves and violet flowers.

2. Cut the avocado, cucumber and cherry tomatoes into pieces.

3. Mix all the ingredients in a bowl.

4. Drizzle salad with olive oil and balsamic vinegar.

5. Add salt and pepper to taste.

6. Finally, add the violet flowers for a delicious floral touch. Enjoy this colorful, fragrant salad with pleasure!

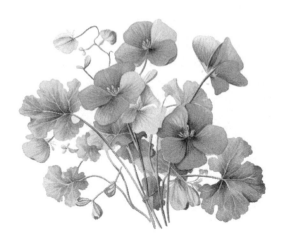

NASTURTIUM
(TROPAEOLUM MAJUS)

THE ORNAMENTAL GARDEN REMEDY

Let's discover nasturtium, an ornamental plant known for its beauty, but also for its many health and culinary benefits.

Nasturtium, originally from South America, was introduced to Europe in the 17th century as an ornamental and medicinal plant. It is renowned for its colorful flowers and water-lily-shaped leaves. Historically, the Incas used nasturtium to disinfect and heal wounds, and it was also valued for its nutritional qualities. It gained popularity in

France in the 18th century, where it was cultivated in gardens for its medicinal and culinary virtues. Nasturtium flowers, leaves and seeds are known for their antimicrobial and expectorant properties, and are rich in vitamins and minerals. They were also used during wartime as a substitute for pepper, hence its nickname of "Peruvian cress".

In the kitchen

Nasturtium is a culinary delight, known for adding **color** and **piquancy** to a variety of dishes. Its edible flowers have a slightly peppery taste, comparable to that of watercress, making salads livelier and more flavorful. The leaves, also edible, are often used as **edible decoration** or added to salads for a spicy touch. Nasturtium seeds can be made into **capers** and are an excellent addition to many dishes. Their pungent, peppery flavor can spice up sauces, meats and vegetables.

Rich in vitamin C, the edible parts of nasturtium are excellent for **boosting the immune system**. In addition to its unique taste, nasturtium offers **antioxidant properties** and health benefits. Its ability to improve **digestion** and fight infection makes this plant both beautiful and useful. Nasturtium's components can also help **improve blood circulation**, making it ideal for people seeking to maintain a balanced, healthy diet. Finally, it's important to consume nasturtium in moderation, as excessive amounts can irritate the urinary and gastrointestinal tracts.

HEALING WITH NASTURTIUM

- For **coughs** and **congestion**, use nasturtium leaves to make a herbal tea. Infuse a tablespoon of leaves in boiling water for 10 minutes, then drink.

- To **disinfect wounds,** apply crushed nasturtium leaves directly to the wound.

- For **urinary tract infections,** use nasturtium regularly as a tea to benefit from its antibacterial properties.

- If you have **skin problems** such as acne or pimples, apply nasturtium juice directly to the skin to help remove impurities and reduce inflammation.

- For **respiratory infections,** inhale steam from a nasturtium decoction to clear the respiratory tract.

- For **vitamin deficiencies,** include nasturtium flowers, leaves and seeds in your diet. They are a rich source of nutrients and vitamin C.

LA CAPUCINE IN THE KITCHEN

Fresh nasturtium salad

INGREDIENTS: A few nasturtium leaves and flowers, 1 cucumber, 2 tomatoes, 100 g feta cheese, 1 tablespoon olive oil, 1 tablespoon balsamic vinegar, salt and pepper.

1. Wash and chop the tomatoes and cucumber. Cut the feta cheese into cubes.

2. Mix the vegetables, feta and nasturtium leaves in a salad bowl.

3. Drizzle with olive oil and balsamic vinegar. Add salt and pepper to taste.

4. Garnish with nasturtium flowers before serving for a colorful, peppery touch. Enjoy this refreshing and nutritious salad!

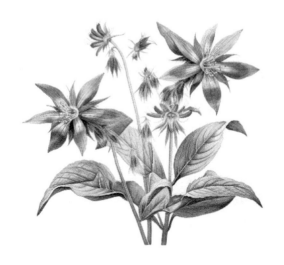

THE BORAGE
(BORAGO OFFICINALIS)

EVERYDAY SERENITY AND WELL-BEING

Let's embark on a journey to the heart of the garden and discover a multi-faceted plant: borage. This starry blue or white flower is a treasure trove of unsuspected benefits and delicate flavors.

Originally from the Middle East, borage has travelled across the continents to become an essential element of European gardens. It has been used since antiquity by the Greeks and Romans for its medicinal and culinary virtues.

It was reputed to bring happiness and relieve stress, which is why it was nicknamed "the plant of good cheer". Known as a medicinal plant, it is used to treat various ailments such as inflammation and skin disorders. Borage also has diuretic and expectorant properties, making it an ally in cases of respiratory and urinary disorders. Leaves and flowers are the most commonly used parts of borage, although they should be consumed in moderation due to their content of pyrrolizidine alkaloids, which are potentially toxic in large quantities.

In the kitchen

Borage is a subtle delight that enriches many dishes. **Rich in vitamins and minerals,** it slips into salads and soups, or serves as a decorative, edible garnish. Its **edible flowers add** a touch of color and make a pleasant condiment, with their cucumber-like flavor. It is particularly appreciated in Mediterranean cuisine, where it enhances pasta and rice dishes. The **young,** tender **leaves** can be eaten raw or cooked, while the older ones are generally used as herbs. **Rich in omega-6 fatty acids,** it contributes to skin and joint health. Its oil, obtained from its seeds, is often used as a **dietary supplement** for its rich gamma-linolenic acid content, known for its **anti-inflammatory** properties. It's a veritable treasure trove of benefits, a concentrate of sweetness and flavor in your dishes, making it easy to combine health and gustatory pleasure. However, due to its alkaloid content, it should be consumed in moderation.

HEALING WITH BORAGE

- To soothe **skin inflammation**, apply a compress of fresh borage leaves to the affected area.

- For **mild stress** or **depression**, drink borage tea. Infuse a teaspoon of dried flowers in a cup of hot water for 5-10 minutes and drink up to three times a day.

- For **coughs** and **respiratory problems**, make a borage syrup. Boil a handful of leaves in 500 ml of water and 500 g of sugar to obtain a syrup. Take one tablespoon three times a day.

- For **joint pain,** massage borage oil directly into the affected areas.

- For **fatigue,** drink borage tea regularly.

- If you suffer from **dermatitis** or **eczema,** apply borage oil to the affected areas to soothe and moisturize the skin.

- To treat **acne,** use borage oil topically on pimples.

BORAGE IN THE KITCHEN

Fresh Borage Salad

INGREDIENTS: 1 handful borage flowers, 150 g baby spinach, 100 g feta cheese, 1 cucumber, olive oil, balsamic vinegar, salt, pepper.

1. Wash and drain baby spinach and borage flowers.

2. Peel and thinly slice the cucumber.

3. Crumble the feta cheese.

4. Mix the spinach, cucumber, feta and borage flowers in a bowl.

5. Season with olive oil, balsamic vinegar, salt and pepper to taste.

6. Mix well and serve chilled. Then enjoy your salad, rich in flavor and health benefits!

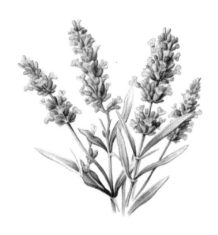

THE LAVENDER
(LAVANDULA)

CALM AND SERENITY IN BLOOM

Lavender is renowned for its enchanting fragrance and soothing properties, offering a unique sensory experience and a journey through the purple fields of the Mediterranean basin.

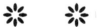

Native to Mediterranean regions, lavender is an aromatic plant that has stood the test of time, conquering the hearts of ancient civilizations such as the Egyptians, Greeks and Romans. These peoples used lavender to perfume their baths and wash their clothes, hence its name derived from the Latin "lavare", meaning to wash. The

Egyptians also used it for mummification. Lavender was synonymous with cleanliness and freshness. In the Middle Ages, lavender gained renown as a remedy for the plague. Over the centuries, its spectrum of uses broadened to include aromatherapy, perfumery, phytotherapy and even cooking. It was considered a panacea for a variety of ailments, including sleep disorders, anxiety and infections. Its purple fields grace the landscapes of Provence, where it has become a symbol of love and tradition. Lavender is prized for its ability to **soothe the mind** and **improve sleep**, and embodies man's eternal quest for tranquility and well-being.

In the kitchen

Lavender, with its floral, slightly sweet aroma, blends harmoniously into contemporary cuisine, especially desserts and pastries. Its dried flowers add a Provencal touch to dishes, while its essential oil, rich in **antiseptic** and **anti-inflammatory properties**, can be incorporated into beverage recipes, conferring not only a unique flavor but also health benefits. Lavender's **calming properties** are particularly sought-after, helping to reduce stress and anxiety while improving sleep. As well as being a popular ingredient in cakes and cookies, lavender is also used to concoct syrups that enhance the flavor of cocktails and lemonades. Its distinctive flavor complements savory dishes, especially white meats and grilled vegetables. However, moderate use is essential, as its powerful taste can quickly dominate a dish. Innovative and versatile, lavender continues to seduce chefs and cooking enthusiasts alike, revealing unexpected flavor combinations and offering an array of health benefits. Its bright floral notes and relaxing benefits make lavender an elegant and benevolent choice in the kitchen, marking every meal with a stamp of serenity.

HEALING WITH LAVENDER

- To soothe **headaches**, mix a few drops of lavender essential oil with a vegetable oil and gently massage the temples.

- For **light burns** or **insect bites**, apply a few drops of lavender essential oil directly to the affected area.

- For **better sleep,** add a few drops of lavender essential oil to your pillow or use an aroma diffuser in your bedroom.

- If you suffer from **dry skin or eczema**, mix a few drops of lavender essential oil with an unscented moisturizer and apply to the skin.

- In case of **anxiety** or **stress**, inhale deeply the aroma of lavender essential oil directly from the bottle or apply diluted to the wrists.

- To **relieve muscle pain,** mix a few drops of lavender essential oil with a massage oil and massage into aching muscles.

- For **skin infections**, apply lavender essential oil diluted in a vegetable oil to the affected area several times a day.

LAVENDER IN THE KITCHEN

Lavender Cookies

INGREDIENTS: 200 g flour, 100 g sugar, 125 g butter, 1 egg, 1 tsp dried lavender flowers, 1 pinch salt.

1. Preheat oven to 180°C. Mix the flour, sugar and salt in a bowl. Add the chopped butter and mix to a sandy dough.

2. Add the egg and mix well. Then add the lavender flowers.

3. Form small balls of dough and place on a baking sheet lined with baking parchment.

4. Bake for approx. 12-15 minutes or until golden brown.

5. Cool on a wire rack and enjoy your lavender cookies!

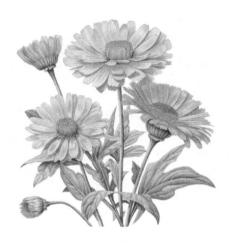

MARIGOLD
(CALENDULA OFFICINALIS)

AN ALLY FOR THE SKIN

Marigold, a flower with sunny hues, is a must-have not only in the garden, but also in phytotherapy, recognized for its many beneficial properties, especially for the skin.

Since ancient times, marigolds have been appreciated for their medicinal virtues and simple beauty. Originally found in the Mediterranean region, it has spread throughout the world. It is often associated with homage to the dead and commemoration in many cultures. Marigold is a symbol of love and affection in popular culture, but beyond its symbolism, it is best known for its benefits in phytotherapy. Marigold is used to treat a variety of skin problems, such as cuts, abrasions and minor burns, and is particularly effective against skin inflammation. It is also renowned for its antifungal and antimicrobial properties, as well as for its ability to stimulate cell regeneration. Internally, it can support digestive health and is used to treat ulcers and inflammation of the gastrointestinal tract. Its dried flowers are often incorporated into herbal teas to take advantage of its benefits.

In the kitchen

Marigolds are also subtle additions to the kitchen, adding color and sweetness to dishes. **Its petals are edible** and can be used to decorate salads, cakes and other dishes. In cooking, marigold is appreciated for its **coloring properties**, used as a substitute for saffron to give dishes a beautiful yellow color. Although not as intensely aromatic as other herbs, it introduces a sweet, earthy nuance to foods. In addition to their visual and gustatory benefits, marigold petals are rich in **flavonoid and antioxidant compounds**, beneficial to overall health. Marigold infusions are delicious, with **soothing properties** and can be consumed to **improve digestion** and **calm gastrointestinal irritations**. Marigold petals are also a choice ingredient for jams and can be incorporated into a variety of baked goods for their unique texture and vibrant color. But before you use them, make sure the marigold flowers are free of pesticides and other chemicals, especially if they're harvested from a garden or public place. In short, marigolds are a beautiful and beneficial addition to both the eye and the palate.

TREATING YOURSELF WITH CARE

- **For skin inflammation**, apply marigold ointment directly to the affected area several times a day.

- **For burns**, use a compress of infused marigold flowers to soothe the skin.

- **For acne and skin irritations,** use a marigold-based soap or lotion daily.

- **For digestive problems,** drink a cup of marigold tea after meals.

- **To soothe a sore throat,** gargle with a chilled infusion of marigold flowers.

- **For cuts and scrapes,** apply marigold gel to promote healing.

- **For fungal infections,** apply a marigold-based cream to the affected area several times a day.

MARIGOLD IN THE KITCHEN

Colorful Marigold Salad

INGREDIENTS: 1 cup marigold petals, 2 cups mixed salad, 1/4 cup walnuts, 1/2 sliced cucumber, 1/4 cup vinaigrette, salt and pepper to taste.

1. Gently wash and dry the marigold petals and greens.

2. Mix the marigold petals with the mixed salad, walnuts and cucumbers in a large bowl.

3. Drizzle the dressing over the salad and toss well to coat all the ingredients.

4. Season with salt and pepper to taste and serve immediately.

5. Enjoy your meal!

This salad is a simple, colorful dish that combines the crunch of walnuts, the freshness of cucumber, and the sweet, earthy notes of marigold petals. The petals not only add color and flavor to the salad, but also a nutritious touch.

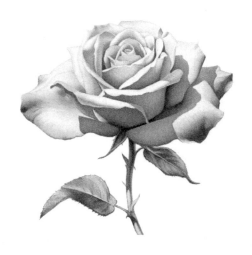

THE ROSE
(ROSA)

FOR SUBTLE, NATURAL BEAUTY

Let's immerse ourselves in the captivating world of the rose, a flower which, beyond its intoxicating fragrance and beauty, holds invaluable virtues and finds its place as much in the kitchen as in cosmetics.

The rose, a universal symbol of love and beauty, has stood the test of time, displaying its petals in a variety of fields, from culinary arts to perfumery. Native to Asia, it has been cultivated for over 5,000 years. The Romans used it in cooking and to decorate their banquets, while the Persians used it for remedies and perfumes. It was during the Middle Ages that the rose spread throughout Europe, where it was first used for its medicinal virtues, before becoming the favorite floral motif of artists and poets. The rose, with its delicate fragrance and many varieties, is a treasure of nature with multiple uses: it purifies, beautifies, heals and, above all, intoxicates our senses with its sublime aroma. The essential oils extracted from its petals have been used for centuries for their soothing, regenerative and anti-inflammatory properties.

In the kitchen

The rose is a culinary jewel that **transforms and subtly enhances** dishes with its delicate fragrance. **In pastries, jams and syrups,** it adds a refined floral note. **Rose-scented sugar** and **rosewater** are popular condiments that blend harmoniously into many recipes, from Oriental baklava to Turkish Turkish Turkish delight. Rose petals, **rich in vitamins and antioxidants**, are not only a delight to the eye but also offer **significant health benefits**, such as anti-inflammatory and soothing properties. Incorporating rose into the kitchen is a fusion of culinary art and health, as it **aids digestion and boosts the immune system**. But not all roses are edible. So it's crucial to opt for organically grown, pesticide-free roses, to enjoy their full flavor and benefits without risk. What's more, the addition of roses lends an exotic twist and a romantic touch to dishes, creating new and memorable culinary experiences.

HEALING WITH ROSE

- To soothe **tired or irritated eyes**, infuse a few rose petals in boiling water, leave to cool and use as an eye compress.

- For **sore throats and hoarseness**, prepare a rose syrup by simmering petals with sugar and water. Take a tablespoon several times a day.

- To **soothe irritated or reddened skin**, apply a lotion made with rosewater. This can also help with **sunburn**.

- If you suffer from **stress or anxiety,** add a few drops of rose essential oil to a diffuser to create a relaxing atmosphere.

- To treat **cuts and abrasions**, apply a few drops of rose essential oil mixed with a carrier oil directly to the affected area.

- For **acne and skin imperfections**, apply a mixture of rose essential oil and vegetable oil locally.

ROSE IN THE KITCHEN

Rose Petal Jam

INGREDIENTS: 100 g edible rose petals, 500 g sugar, juice of 2 lemons, 500 ml water.

1. Gently wash and drain the rose petals.

2. In a saucepan, add the rose petals, sugar, water and lemon juice.

3. Bring the mixture to the boil, then reduce heat and simmer for 20-30 minutes, or until thickened.

4. Once the jam is ready, let it cool, then transfer to sterilized jars and close the lids tightly.

5. Enjoy this rose petal jam on toast or pancakes, or add it to pastries for a subtle, exquisite floral taste.

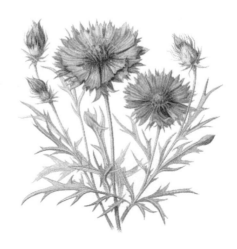

LE CORNFLOWER
(CENTAUREA CYANUS)

MEDICINAL AND CULINARY BEAUTY

Let's embark on a new botanical journey by discovering the cornflower, a delicate flower in shades of blue, renowned for its therapeutic virtues and varied culinary uses.

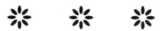

Native to the Near East, cornflowers have been valued for their medicinal properties since Antiquity. Greeks and Romans used it to soothe eye and skin ailments. The flower, symbolizing gentleness, also featured in medieval poetry, where it was a metaphor for tender love. In the Middle Ages, ladies applied it to their eyelids to soothe tired eyes. This practice gave rise to its popular name of "eyeglass breaker". The cornflower has survived the centuries and continues to be one of the most appreciated medicinal and culinary plants. Because of its many virtues, it is often used in herbal teas to relieve digestive problems and eye inflammation. It is also an excellent remedy for skin infections. Natural skincare enthusiasts cherish cornflower for their soothing, anti-inflammatory properties, which are highly beneficial for sensitive, irritated skin.

In the kitchen

Cornflower, with their edible petals, embellish and perfume dishes with a **gentle flavor**. Rich in **antioxidants** and **anti-inflammatory** compounds, it blends well in salads, desserts and drinks, giving a vibrant hue and a subtle sweet note. Its petals can be used to prepare syrups, jams and liqueurs, adding a floral touch to your culinary creations. Cornflowers **are** also a treasure trove of health benefits. Rich in vitamins and minerals, it helps **fight inflammation** and **improve digestion**. It is frequently added to herbal tea blends for its **soothing** and **detoxifying** properties. Finally, in desserts, cornflower, with their bluish hues, offer a colorful, delicate touch, while enhancing sweet flavors with their subtle fragrance. Whether in cakes, pastries or ice creams, incorporating cornflower adds a gastronomic dimension that delights lovers of floral flavors. Integrating cornflower into the kitchen means not only enjoying their exquisite flavor, but also benefiting from their nutritional attributes, contributing to a balanced and tasty diet.

HEALING WITH CORNFLOWER

- To **soothe tired or irritated eyes**, infuse a tablespoon of dried cornflowers in 250 ml of boiling water for 10 minutes, strain and use as compresses.

- For **sore throats**, make an infusion with a teaspoon of dried flowers in a cup of hot water and gargle several times a day.

- For **skin irritations**, apply a compress soaked in cornflower decoction to the affected area.

- To **treat mouth inflammation**, rinse your mouth with an infusion of cornflower flowers three times a day.

- To **improve digestion,** drink a cup of cornflower infusion after meals.

- If you have **cuts or abrasions,** apply cornflower ointment to **promote healing**.

- For **dry or irritated skin,** use cornflower oil as a moisturizer.

CORNFLOWER IN THE KITCHEN

*Cornflower **jelly***

INGREDIENTS: 3 cups fresh or dried cornflower flowers, 2 cups water, 2 cups sugar, 1 sachet pectin.

1. Infuse the cornflower in boiling water for about 10 minutes, then strain to remove the flowers.

2. Mix the liquid with the pectin and bring to the boil.

3. Add the sugar and stir until completely dissolved.

4. Continue boiling for 2 minutes.

5. Pour the jelly into sterilized jars and leave to cool.

6. Once cooled, cornflower jelly is ready to enjoy on toast or pancakes, or to sweeten and flavour tea or yoghurt!

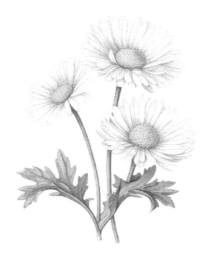

DAISY
(BELLIS PERENNIS)

THE LITTLE GARDEN STAR

Let's immerse ourselves in the discreet charm of daisies, the little white flowers that adorn our gardens and lawns, revealing their often overlooked beauty and benefits.

Known for its pretty little white flowers with yellow hearts, the daisy, a modest inhabitant of our gardens, is endowed with remarkable properties. A member of the

Asteraceae family, it has been renowned since Antiquity for its many medicinal virtues. The Romans used daisy to beautify and tone the skin, while the ancient Greeks appreciated it for its anti-inflammatory benefits. In the Middle Ages, it was eaten in salads and used as a remedy for skin ailments and respiratory disorders. The daisy, which flowers almost all year round, is also known for its diuretic and depurative properties, making it an ideal ally for cleansing the body.

In the kitchen

The **daisy is** more than just a garden ornament. The flowers, fresh or dried, can be added to salads and dishes, offering a delicate, decorative touch. In addition to their aesthetic appeal, daisies provide **numerous health benefits**, being rich in antioxidants and anti-inflammatory compounds. They can also be infused to make sweet and beneficial herbal teas, known to **improve digestion** and **boost the immune system**. In the kitchen, you can make daisy syrups and jams which, in addition to their delicate, floral flavours, help to **improve skin health** and **balance the respiratory system**. Use these syrups and jams to sweeten drinks and pastries, or as a base for floral vinaigrettes. Similarly, daisy-infused oil can be used as a **seasoning**, adding not only flavor to your dishes but also **nutritional and therapeutic value**. By incorporating daisy into your meals, you add a touch of floral flavor while enjoying its multiple health benefits. It's a delicious and original way to combine gustatory pleasure and well-being.

HEALING WITH DAISIES

- To **soothe the skin**, apply daisy flowers infused in oil to irritated areas.

- For **coughs and sore throats,** infuse the flowers in hot water and drink this mild tea several times a day.

- To relieve **joint pain**, prepare a poultice with crushed fresh flowers and apply to painful areas.

- For **respiratory problems,** inhale the aroma of a decoction of daisy flowers to help clear the airways.

- If you have **digestive problems,** drink daisy tea to aid digestion and soothe the digestive system.

- For **skin disorders** such as acne, apply an infusion of cooled daisy as a compress to the skin.

- For **light cuts or wounds**, apply fresh daisy juice for its antiseptic properties.

DAISY IN THE KITCHEN

Spring Salad with Daisy

INGREDIENTS: 1 handful daisy flowers, 100 g baby spinach, 50 g fresh goat's cheese, 50 g walnuts, 1 tbsp olive oil, 1 tsp balsamic vinegar, salt and pepper.

1. Gently wash and dry the daisy flowers and baby spinach shoots.

2. In a bowl, combine the spinach, crumbled goat's cheese and chopped walnuts.

3. Drizzle with olive oil and balsamic vinegar, and season to taste.

4. Mix gently and garnish with the daisy flowers just before serving.

5. Enjoy this fresh, crunchy salad with subtle floral notes!

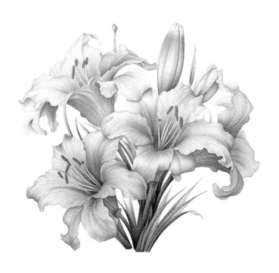

DAYLILY
(HEMEROCALLIS)

EPHEMERAL BEAUTY AND LASTING BENEFITS

Hemerocallis, nicknamed "Beauty for a Day", not only dazzles with its luminous flowers, but also offers a multitude of culinary and therapeutic benefits that last well beyond its ephemeral bloom.

Hemerocallis has been appreciated for centuries, especially in East Asia where it originated. Known for its majestic, ephemeral flowers, this hardy perennial has crossed the ages and continents, becoming naturalized in many parts of the world. The Chinese, Japanese and

Koreans traditionally used Hemerocallis for its medicinal properties, notably its diuretic and laxative effects. As well as being a remedy, it has long served as an ornamental plant in Asian gardens, symbolizing fleeting beauty and rebirth. Hemerocallis was introduced to Europe around the 16th century, and was adopted to beautify gardens and for the medicinal properties of its flowers, leaves and roots. The flowers are often used in traditional cooking for their delicate, sweet flavors and are rich in vitamins and minerals.

In the kitchen

Hemerocallis is a subtle and nutritious delight in modern cooking. The **edible flowers** add a touch of color and a uniquely sweet flavor to salads and desserts. The buds can be cooked like greens, adding a crisp, fresh note. The flowers' **rich vitamin and mineral content** contributes to nutritional balance, while offering **antioxidant** properties that fight free radicals. Hemerocallis are also appreciated for their ability to provide **satiety** and **balance**, making them ideal for a variety of diets. **In traditional medicine,** Daylilies are used to treat insomnia and inflammation. The roots are renowned for their **diuretic** and **laxative properties**, offering a natural remedy for a variety of digestive disorders. Hemerocallis' versatility and nutritional value make it invaluable in vegetarian and vegan cooking, and it can be used to add depth of flavor and a touch of color to many dishes, from the simple to the sophisticated. Be careful, however, to consume it in moderate quantities, as some varieties can have a laxative effect if eaten in large quantities.

TREATMENT WITH DAYLILY

- For **digestive disorders,** infuse a few dried petals in boiling water for 10 minutes. Strain and drink this infusion up to twice a day.

- For **insomnia,** drink an infusion of fresh flowers to benefit from their relaxing, sleep-inducing properties.

- If you suffer from **constipation,** raw or cooked flowers can be consumed as a natural remedy due to their mild **laxative** properties.

- To soothe **skin inflammation**, apply a poultice of fresh petals directly to the affected area.

- For **water retention,** use a decoction of the roots as a natural diuretic.

- To relieve **sore throats,** gargle with an infusion of Hemerocallis petals two or three times a day.

- If you have **light burns or cuts**, apply the fresh juice of the plant directly to the wound for accelerated healing.

DAYLILY IN THE KITCHEN

Hemerocallis Salad with Honey Vinaigrette

INGREDIENTS: 6 fresh Hemerocallis flowers, 100 g arugula, 50 g walnuts, 1 tbsp honey, 2 tbsp balsamic vinegar, 4 tbsp olive oil, salt, pepper.

1. Gently wash and dry the Hemerocallis flowers, then separate the petals.

2. Mix the arugula, Hemerocallis petals and walnuts in a salad bowl.

3. For the vinaigrette, combine the honey, balsamic vinegar, olive oil, salt and pepper in a small bowl.

4. Pour the vinaigrette over the salad, toss gently and serve immediately. Enjoy this crunchy, colorful salad!

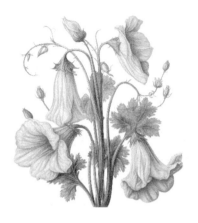

ZUCCHINI FLOWERS
(CUCURBITA PEPO)

A BURST OF FLAVOUR ON THE PLATE

Let's discover the delicate and delicious zucchini flower, a culinary treasure straight from the kitchen garden, rich in flavor and endowed with interesting nutritional and medicinal properties.

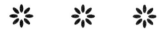

Native to the tropical regions of South America, the zucchini, and hence its flower, has been an essential element of Mediterranean cuisine since the Renaissance. Today, zucchini flowers are prized for their subtle flavor and tender texture, and are often used in Italian and French cuisine to create sumptuous and artistic dishes. They can be stuffed, fried or used as a garnish, offering delicate flavor and vibrant color to dishes. Historically, in addition to their culinary use, these flowers were used for their medicinal properties, notably to treat various ailments such as inflammation and skin irritation.

In the kitchen

Zucchini blossom is a summertime culinary staple, particularly appreciated for its **sweetness and delicate texture**. It goes wonderfully well with a multitude of flavors and textures. In the kitchen, they are often **stuffed with** cheese and herbs, then **fried to a** crisp. Their subtle flavor and tender texture add a **unique dimension to** the dishes in which they are incorporated. **Rich in vitamins A and C,** these flowers are also a nutritional asset. They are also **low in calories**, making them ideal for those watching their weight.

They can also be used to prepare summer salads, adding a colorful **floral touch.** Zucchini flowers contain **lutein**, an antioxidant important for eye health. They also have **anti-inflammatory** and **diuretic** properties, and are used in traditional medicine to treat a variety of ailments, including skin disorders and inflammation. In short, zucchini flowers are not only a delight for the palate, but also a source of health benefits. So, the next time you find yourself with zucchini flowers, don't hesitate to incorporate them into your cooking to add a touch of color, flavor and nutrition to your dishes.

HEALING WITH ZUCCHINI FLOWER

- For **skin irritations**, you can make an infusion of zucchini flowers. Apply this infusion gently to the irritated area.

- For **digestive problems,** drink an infusion of zucchini flowers to help soothe the digestive system.

- To relieve **inflammation,** regularly incorporate zucchini flowers into your diet, as they have anti-inflammatory properties.

- In cases of **water retention,** zucchini flowers can be used for their diuretic properties, helping to eliminate excess water from the body.

- For **eyesight problems**, increase your consumption of zucchini flowers, which are rich in lutein, beneficial for eye health.

- To improve **skin health**, apply a paste made from crushed zucchini flowers to the skin to take advantage of their antioxidant properties.

ZUCCHINI FLOWERS IN THE KITCHEN

Zucchini flower fritters

INGREDIENTS: 12 zucchini flowers, 100 g flour, 1 egg, 150 ml milk, 1 pinch salt, frying oil.

1. Mix flour, egg, milk and salt in a bowl until smooth.

2. Gently wash the zucchini flowers and pat dry with kitchen paper.

3. Heat the oil in a frying pan. Dip each flower in the batter and fry until golden.

4. Drain the doughnuts on kitchen paper and serve hot, with a dash of salt if desired. Enjoy!

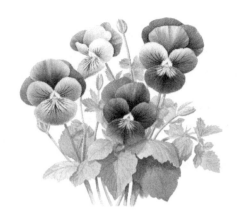

THE PANSY
(VIOLA X WITTROCKIANA)

A SYMBOL OF REMEMBRANCE AND LOVE

Let's discover a plant that, although a picturesque symbol of remembrance and love, also has benefits that are often overlooked: the pansy, a flower with a rich history and culinary and medicinal virtues.

   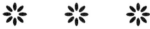

Known for its charming face and bright colors, the pansy is a flower that has stood the test of time, symbolizing love and memory. Native to Europe and Asia, this flower has been cultivated and hybridized, giving rise to a multitude of varieties and colors. Pansies are appreciated for their beauty and used in many gardens around the world, but they were once valued for their medicinal properties, notably to treat skin and respiratory ailments. Pansy was also a source of spiritual comfort in folk traditions, often associated with lost love and remembrance. The ancient Greeks and Romans used pansies as a symbol of eternal love, placing them on the altars of love gods such as Aphrodite and Eros. In the Middle Ages, they were considered a love charm and a means of transmitting secret messages between lovers.

In the kitchen

Not only is the pansy a visually pleasing flower, it is also edible and **rich in vitamins and minerals.** It adds a colorful, delicate touch to dishes, while offering **anti-inflammatory and diuretic properties.** It can be used to garnish salads and desserts, or to create pleasant and beneficial infusions. Pansies are **rich in flavonoids,** known for their antioxidant properties, and can therefore help boost the immune system and combat free radicals in the body. In traditional medicine, pansies are used to treat a variety of ailments, such as eczema and asthma. They are also known to **relieve the symptoms of respiratory disorders.** Pansy infusions are particularly useful in winter, when the immune system may need a boost. Although pansies are generally considered safe to consume, it's always advisable to use them in moderation, and to check for allergies beforehand. The delicacy and color diversity of pansies make them ideal for edible decoration, adding a touch of elegance and subtle aroma to your dishes.

HEALING WITH PANSY

- To soothe **skin ailments**, infuse a handful of pansy flowers in boiling water and use the water to cleanse the affected skin.

- For **coughs and sore throats**, prepare an herbal tea by infusing pansy flowers in hot water. Drink this infusion up to three times a day.

- **For breathing** problems **and asthma,** inhale steam from a pansy decoction to soothe the respiratory tract.

- If you suffer from **urinary or kidney problems**, drink an infusion of pansy regularly for its diuretic properties.

- For **eye irritations**, use an infusion of cooled pansy as a compress to soothe the eyes.

- For **eczema,** apply a paste made from crushed pansy flowers and a little water to the affected areas.

- To **boost the immune system,** drink pansy infusions regularly.

PANSY IN THE KITCHEN

Pansy Fruit Salad

INGREDIENTS: 1 cup sliced strawberries, 1 cup cubed pineapple, 1 cup grapes, 1 cup cubed melon, a handful of edible pansy flowers.

1. Mix all the fruit in a large bowl.
2. Garnish with pansy flowers.
3. If desired, drizzle with honey or agave syrup for a sweet touch.
4. Refrigerate the salad for an hour before serving to allow the flavours to blend.
5. Serve chilled and enjoy this fruity, flowery salad!

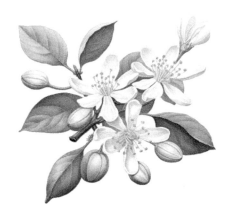

THE LINDEN TREE
(TILIA)

A SOOTHING ALLY FOR OUR NIGHTS

Lime, known for its pleasant fragrance and soothing properties, is a must for fans of herbal teas and natural remedies, offering a journey through medicinal traditions.

The Linden tree, also called Lime trees, sacred to many cultures, has a long and rich history in the field of natural medicine. It grows in temperate regions of the northern hemisphere, notably in Europe and Asia. The Celts saw the lime tree as a symbol of love and peace, and in ancient

Greece it was dedicated to the goddess Aphrodite. Linden's calming and relaxing properties were already known to the Romans, who used it to soothe nerves and promote sleep. In the Middle Ages, lime was associated with protection and love, and it was common to meet under a lime tree to resolve conflicts. Today, lime is still appreciated for its soothing benefits and its role in relieving stress and anxiety, treating colds and promoting restful sleep. Linden is also known for its anti-inflammatory and antispasmodic properties, useful for headaches and difficult digestion.

In the kitchen

Lime has a place in our kitchens, mainly in the form of delicious, **soothing** herbal teas. It can also be used to flavor sweet and savory dishes. Linden flowers can be added to salads for a floral touch or used to infuse syrups and liqueurs. Linden's **relaxing** and **anti-inflammatory** properties make it a valuable ally for calming the digestive system, **reducing anxiety** and **improving sleep**. In Ayurveda, linden is valued for its action on doshas balance, and is considered beneficial for calming Vata and Kapha.

Linden can also enrich desserts, creams and cakes, adding a subtle, fragrant floral note. In addition to its presence in cooking, linden is also appreciated for its health benefits, being rich in flavonoids, antioxidant compounds. That's why linden infusion is often consumed to **relieve headaches**, **calm nerves** and **aid digestion**. People with sleep problems can benefit from its **sedative** properties by drinking a cup of linden tea before bedtime. Be careful, however, not to overuse it, as excessive consumption can lead to heart problems.

HEALING WITH LIME BLOSSOM

- For **sleep disorders**, infuse a tablespoon of dried lime blossom in a cup of boiling water for 10 minutes. Drink this infusion before going to bed.

- To **soothe nerves**, make an herbal tea by infusing 2 tablespoons of dried flowers in 500 ml of boiling water for 10 minutes. Drink 2 to 3 cups a day.

- If you suffer from **headaches,** apply a compress soaked in linden tea to your forehead.

- To **relieve colds,** inhale the vapors from a decoction of linden blossoms.

- For **difficult digestion,** drink linden tea after meals.

- For **menstrual pain,** drink one to two cups of linden tea a day during your period.

- If you have **skin problems** such as abcesses or inflammation, apply a lime blossom poultice locally.

LINDEN IN THE KITCHEN

Lime shortbread

INGREDIENTS: 125g butter, 100g sugar, 1 egg, 200g flour, 1 pinch salt, 1 tablespoon dried lime blossom, finely chopped.

1. Preheat oven to 180°C (gas mark 6).

2. Mix butter and sugar until creamy.

3. Add the egg, then the flour, salt and chopped lime blossom.

4. Knead lightly and form into a ball.

5. On a floured work surface, roll out the dough to a thickness of 5 mm and cut out shapes with a cookie cutter.

6. Place the shortbread on a baking tray lined with baking paper and bake for 10 to 12 minutes, or until golden brown.

7. Leave to cool and enjoy!

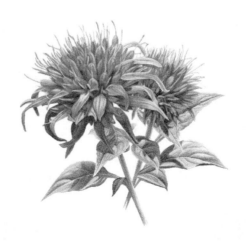

THE MONARDE
(MONARDA)

A JEWEL OF THE AROMATIC GARDEN

Let's discover Monarde, a multi-faceted ornamental plant native to North America, where it is a delight for butterflies, bees and, of course, gardeners.

Monarde, also known as bergamot, is a perennial plant belonging to the Lamiaceae family. It is famous for its flamboyant flowers and aromatic leaves. Native Americans used Monarde to treat a variety of ailments, including respiratory infections and digestive problems. Monarde leaves, rich in thymol, have antiseptic properties.

Introduced to Europe in the 17th century, it is appreciated in cooking for its bergamot-like aroma. There are many varieties of Monarde, and they are appreciated for their ease of cultivation, being resistant to many pests and diseases. They are planted in gardens as much for their decorative qualities as for their medicinal and culinary properties.

In the kitchen

Monarde is a wonderful addition to the culinary garden. **Its fragrant leaves** can be used fresh or dried as a condiment, adding a lemony, spicy note to salads, soups and desserts. **Rich in thymol**, Monarde has **antiseptic and antifungal properties**. It is therefore an excellent natural preservative for culinary preparations. Monarde's **edible flowers** can be used to decorate dishes and salads. They can also be crystallized to decorate cakes, or incorporated into syrups and liqueurs to give them a unique flavor. **As an infusion,** Monarde aids digestion and is used as a remedy for colds, sore throats and mouth infections, thanks to its **antibacterial properties**. It is also valued for **stimulating blood circulation and relieving menstrual disorders**. In short, Monarde is not only an asset to your garden, but also an invaluable ally in your kitchen and first-aid kit, making dishes delicious and offering a panoply of health benefits. Monarde should be used in moderation in the kitchen, however, as its taste is quite powerful and can overpower other flavors if used in large quantities.

TREATMENT WITH MONARDA

- To soothe **sore throats,** infuse a few Monarde leaves in hot water and gargle with the infusion several times a day.

- If you suffer from **digestive problems**, make an herbal tea with a handful of fresh Monarde leaves and drink it after meals.

- For **skin problems such as acne,** apply a compress soaked in Monarde decoction to the affected areas.

- In case of a **cold or nasal congestion**, inhale the vapors from an infusion of Monarde to clear the respiratory tract.

- For **mouth infections,** use a decoction of Monarde as a mouthwash several times a day.

- If you have tension **headaches,** massage your temples with a few drops of Monarde essential oil diluted in a carrier oil.

- To relieve **menstrual pain,** drink a cup of Monarde tea two or three times a day during your period.

MONARDE IN THE KITCHEN

Summer Salad with Monarde

INGREDIENTS: 150 g baby lettuce, 6 Monarde flowers, 50 g pine nuts, 50 g feta cheese, 1 tablespoon olive oil, 1 tablespoon balsamic vinegar, salt and pepper.

1. Wash and spin-dry the lettuce shoots and Monarde flowers.

2. In a bowl, combine the baby greens, crumbled Monarde flowers, pine nuts and diced feta cheese.

3. In a small bowl, combine the olive oil and balsamic vinegar. Season to taste with salt and pepper.

4. Pour the vinaigrette over the salad and toss gently.

5. Serve immediately and enjoy the unique flavor of Monarde in this refreshing summer salad.

PART II: TROPICAL AND EXOTIC EDIBLE FLOWERS

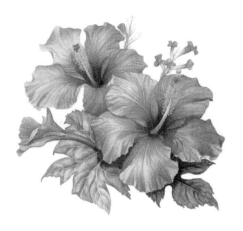

HIBISCUS
(HIBISCUS ROSA-SINENSIS)

A BURST OF FLAVOR AND COLOR

Let's immerse ourselves in the vibrant, colorful world of the hibiscus, an exotic flower known for its distinctive flavors and many medicinal properties, a true star of the tropics.

Native to the warmer regions of Asia and Africa, the hibiscus has a rich and diverse history. This ornamental plant, with its large, bright flowers, has been cultivated since ancient times for its many medicinal and culinary properties. From Egyptian pharaohs to Chinese emperors, many have benefited from its benefits. The Egyptians used it to regulate body temperature and treat heart and nervous disorders. In China, it was mainly used as an offering during spiritual ceremonies. Hibiscus was introduced to Europe in the 12th century by the Moors and quickly gained popularity for its beauty and medicinal virtues. Today, it is world-renowned for its distinctive taste and multiple health benefits. The various parts of the plant are used in traditional medicine to treat conditions such as hypertension, respiratory infections and digestive disorders. Hibiscus is also a powerful cultural symbol, representing beauty and fragility in many cultures around the world.

In the kitchen

Hibiscus occupies a prominent place in world cuisine, bringing a **burst of flavor and color** to dishes and beverages. **Rich in vitamins, minerals and antioxidants**, it is not only nutritious but also therapeutic. Dried hibiscus flowers are often used to make tangy herbal teas, reputed to **lower blood pressure** and **improve digestive health**. They can also be used to make syrups, jams and chutneys, adding a touch of color and a uniquely tangy taste. **A powerful antioxidant**, hibiscus helps **combat oxidative stress and inflammation**, contributing to the prevention of many chronic diseases. It's also a **natural diuretic**, helping the body to eliminate excess fluids and salts. But beware of excessive consumption, as it can affect estrogen levels in the body. In cooking, it is also used as a natural colorant, giving a vibrant red hue to dishes. Chefs around the world are using hibiscus to create visually appealing and nutritionally balanced dishes, exploring its versatility in both savory and sweet preparations, making this exotic flower a must-have in global gastronomy.

HEALING WITH HIBISCUS

- For **high blood pressure,** infuse a few dried hibiscus flowers in boiling water for 5 to 10 minutes. Drink twice a day.

- For **digestive problems,** take a teaspoon of dried hibiscus flowers, infuse in a cup of hot water for 5 minutes and drink before meals.

- For **skin infections**, make a paste with crushed hibiscus flowers and water. Apply to the affected area and leave on for 15-20 minutes.

- To **improve hair health**, use a hibiscus decoction as a final rinse after shampooing. It helps strengthen roots and leaves hair silky.

- For **sore throats,** gargle with a warm infusion of hibiscus several times a day.

- If you suffer from **headaches,** apply compresses of warm hibiscus infusion to the forehead.

- To **combat insomnia,** drink a cup of hibiscus tea before bedtime.

HIBISCUS IN THE KITCHEN

Hibiscus sorbet

INGREDIENTS: 200 g sugar, 1 liter water, 10 dried hibiscus flowers, juice of one lemon.

1. Bring the water to the boil, add the sugar and stir until dissolved.

2. Add the dried hibiscus flowers, remove from the heat, cover and leave to infuse for around 30 minutes.

3. Strain the mixture to remove the flowers, then add the lemon juice.

4. Allow the mixture to cool completely, then pour into an ice-cream maker.

5. Turn into sorbet according to your machine's instructions.

6. Once ready, serve the sorbet in bowls and enjoy chilled!

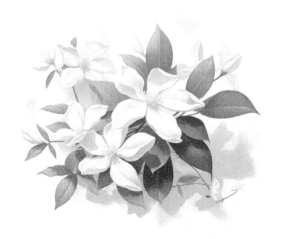

JASMINE
(JASMINUM)

AN INTOXICATING AND HEALING FRAGRANCE

Let's enter the aromatic world of jasmine, an exquisite flower highly prized not only for its bewitching fragrance but also for its many therapeutic properties.

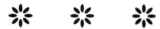

Originally from the Himalayas and Persia, jasmine traveled throughout Asia and the Middle East before settling in China and the rest of the world. It has been cultivated for its fragrant flowers for thousands of years. Jasmine was used by Persian kings to create perfumes and flavored beverages, while the Chinese used it to scent their rooms and clothes. In India, it is considered sacred and used for religious ceremonies and weddings. Jasmine also has a place in Greek and Roman mythology, where it is associated with love and beauty. It arrived in Europe in the 16th century, and soon found its way into French perfumery. Today, jasmine is synonymous with elegance and refinement, and continues to seduce with its distinctive fragrance and medicinal properties.

In the kitchen

Jasmine enhances many culinary preparations, particularly in Asian cuisine. It is often used to flavour tea, producing a sweet, floral and refreshing drink. **An antioxidant**, jasmine tea has **relaxing properties** and can **reduce stress**. It is rich in **polyphenols**, which can help **reduce the risk of heart disease**. Jasmine is also used in desserts, such as tapioca pearls with coconut milk and jasmine, adding a subtle, delicate floral touch. In addition to its culinary applications, jasmine essential oil, extracted from its flowers, has **soothing and anti-inflammatory properties**. In aromatherapy, jasmine oil is used to **treat depression, anxiety, stress and insomnia**. This essential oil is also **anti-catarrhal** and **expectorant**, beneficial for respiratory ailments. Be careful, however, to use it diluted to avoid skin reactions. So jasmine is much more than an intoxicatingly fragrant flower; it's a versatile ingredient that can enhance our general well-being, through both its gustatory and therapeutic properties.

HEALING WITH JASMINE

- To **soothe anxiety** and **reduce stress**, prepare a cup of jasmine tea. Steep a handful of dried jasmine flowers in hot water for 5 to 10 minutes. Drink this tea once or twice a day.

- To **improve sleep,** put a few drops of jasmine essential oil on your pillow or use an essential oil diffuser in your bedroom.

- For **dry or irritated skin,** mix a few drops of jasmine essential oil with coconut oil and apply to the skin.

- To **relieve menstrual cramps**, gently massage your abdomen with a few drops of jasmine essential oil mixed with a carrier oil such as sweet almond oil.

- For **coughs and colds,** inhale steam from boiling water with a few drops of jasmine essential oil added.

- To treat **scars and** skin **imperfections**, apply a mixture of jasmine essential oil and jojoba oil locally.

- For **headaches,** inhale deeply the aroma of jasmine essential oil or massage a few drops onto your temples.

JASMINE IN THE KITCHEN

Jasmine and Honey Tea

INGREDIENTS: 1 tablespoon dried jasmine flowers, 1 tablespoon green tea, 1 tablespoon honey, 500 ml water.

1. Bring the water to the boil and pour over the green tea and jasmine flowers.

2. Leave to infuse for 5 minutes, then strain to remove leaves and flowers.

3. Add honey to taste and stir well until honey is dissolved.

4. Serve hot and enjoy this sweet, aromatic tea, renowned for its relaxing and soothing properties.

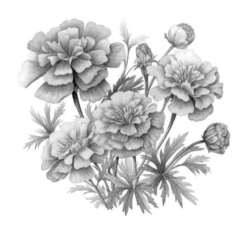

TAGETE
(TAGETES)

SUNSHINE IN THE KITCHEN AND GARDEN

Let's plunge into the world of plants with the tagetes, a remarkable flower known for its vivid colors and varied uses, oscillating between ornamental, culinary and natural care.

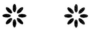

Tagetes, commonly known as "marigolds", are native to Central America, Mexico to be precise. They were introduced to Europe in the 16th century by Spanish explorers. Recognized by their bright yellow or orange flowers, they are mainly used as ornamental plants, bringing life and color to gardens and balconies. However, their use doesn't stop at ornamentation. In Mesoamerican cultures, tagetes had a significant place, both culinary and medicinal. It was used to treat digestive, respiratory and skin disorders. Tagetes petals, with their slightly lemony, spicy taste, were eaten in salads or used as food coloring. These flowers were also incorporated into various rituals and ceremonies, symbolizing life and fertility.

In the kitchen

Tagetes stand out in the kitchen for their unique taste and remarkable **culinary properties. Tagetes** petals can **enhance the flavors of** salads, soups and even desserts, adding a zesty, peppery touch. **Rich in antioxidants**, these flowers contribute to overall health, helping to fight free radicals in the body. They have **digestive properties**, aiding digestion and helping to soothe gastrointestinal disorders. In addition to its health benefits, tagetes also serves as a **natural** food **coloring agent**, providing an attractive yellow-orange hue. The use of this flower in cooking is not limited to its fresh form. Dried, the petals can be used as a **spice or aromatic herb**, adding a distinctive note to dishes and infusions. It's an exceptional way to add not only color but also a new gustatory dimension to your preparations, while enjoying its **health benefits**. By incorporating tagetes into your cooking, you bring a vibrant and beneficial visual and gustatory aspect, making every dish a sensory and nutritional delight.

HEALING WITH TAGETES

- To relieve **skin inflammation**, apply a paste made from crushed tagetes petals and a little water directly to the affected area.

- For **digestive problems**, infuse a teaspoon of dried petals in a cup of boiling water for 5-10 minutes and drink up to three times a day.

- For **eye conditions,** use tagetes infusion as an eyewash to help reduce inflammation and irritation.

- For **skin infections**, apply a few drops of Tagetes essential oil diluted in a carrier oil directly to the affected area.

- For **cuts and scratches,** tagetes petals can be crushed and applied directly for their antiseptic properties.

- If you suffer from **painful periods,** drinking tagetes infusion can help relieve cramps.

- For **respiratory problems**, inhale the aroma of tagetes essential oil to clear the airways.

TAGETES IN THE KITCHEN

Summer salad with Tagetes

INGREDIENTS: 1 cup tagetes petals, 200 g lettuce, 100 g cherry tomatoes, 50 g cucumber, 1 avocado, juice of 1 lemon, 2 tbsp olive oil, salt and pepper.

1. Wash and dry the tagetes petals and vegetables.

2. Chop the lettuce, cherry tomatoes, cucumber and avocado.

3. Mix the tagetes petals with the vegetables in a large bowl.

4. Drizzle with lemon juice and olive oil, then season with salt and pepper to taste.

5. Toss well before serving. Enjoy this fresh, fragrant salad that will delight your senses and add an original touch to your meal.

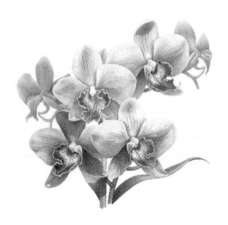

THE ORCHID
(ORCHIDACEAE)

THE QUEEN OF TROPICAL FLOWERS

Let's discover the orchid, the queen of tropical flowers which, beyond its beauty, hides astonishing culinary and medicinal properties, often unknown to the general public.

The orchid, with its varied shapes and colors, is one of the world's largest flower families, comprising thousands of species on almost every continent. Its name comes from the Greek "Orkhis", referring to the shape of its tubers. Historically, orchids were primarily recognized for their beauty and were often associated with lust and sensuality in different cultures. However, there is also a long history of orchid use in traditional medicine in China, India and other parts of Asia. The Vanilla genus, for example, also belongs to the orchid family and is famous for its use in cooking. Orchids are cultivated for their flowers, but some species are also used for their medicinal and nutritional properties. Orchids symbolize beauty, love and strength in many cultures, and despite their frequent association with tropical climates, they can be found in a variety of habitats, including forests, mountains and meadows.

In the kitchen

The **orchid** is not just a decorative flower. It plays an essential role in our cuisine, in particular the **Vanilla** genus, which produces vanilla, an ingredient much appreciated in the world of patisserie for its **unique aroma**. Vanilla is used to flavor many sweet dishes and some savory ones. But did you know that other orchid species are also **edible**, and can be eaten as vegetables or used to make flavored drinks? **Salep**, a flour made from the tubers of certain orchid species, is a popular drink in the Middle East and is known for its **nutritive and digestive properties**. It is rich in mucilage, renowned for its **soothing** effect on the digestive system. Other orchid species are used in traditional Asian medicine for their **anti-inflammatory and antioxidant properties**. Their uses are diverse and varied, ranging from the preparation of **syrups** and **elixirs** to delicate dishes, illustrating the richness of this exceptional floral family. But not all orchids are edible, and some can be toxic. It is therefore essential to be familiar with the species before using them in cooking.

HEALING WITH ORCHIDS

- To soothe **coughs** and **sore throats**, make a decoction with dried orchid petals. Boil a cup of water and add a tablespoon of orchid petals. Leave to infuse for 10 minutes, strain and drink twice a day.

- In cases of **stress** or **anxiety,** orchid tea can have a relaxing effect. Infuse orchid blossoms in hot water for a few minutes, and drink this soothing beverage as needed.

- For **skin problems** such as acne, create a face mask with orchid powder and water. Apply this mixture to your face and leave on for 20 minutes before rinsing off with lukewarm water.

- If you have **digestive problems,** drink orchid tea to stimulate digestion and relieve stomach upset.

ORCHIDS IN THE KITCHEN

Vanilla Ice Cream with Orchid Petals

INGREDIENTS: 500 ml single cream, 250 ml milk, 150 g sugar, 1 vanilla pod, 1 tablespoon edible orchid petals.

1. Split the vanilla pod in half and scrape out the seeds. Place the seeds and vanilla pod in a saucepan with the milk and cream, and bring to the boil.

2. In a bowl, mix the sugar and egg yolks until the mixture whitens.

3. Pour the hot mixture over the egg and sugar mixture, stirring constantly.

4. Return the mixture to the pan and cook over a low heat until the cream coats the spoon.

5. Strain the custard and leave to cool.

6. Once the cream has cooled, ice it in an ice-cream maker according to the manufacturer's instructions.

7. Add the chopped orchid petals as the ice cream begins to set. Once the ice cream is ready, serve and enjoy!

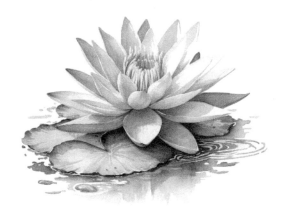

WATER LILIES
(NYMPHAEA)

A SYMBOL OF PURITY AND TRANQUILLITY

Dive into the mysterious world of aquatic plants with the water lily, an ethereal flower and symbol of purity and serenity, often associated with the imagery of Zen gardens and peaceful ponds.

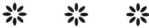

The water lily, a majestic aquatic flower, is often depicted in art and literature as a symbol of purity, beauty and tranquility. It grows in calm waters, embellishing ponds and lakes with its delicate floating flowers. The Nymphaea genus includes many species and varieties, with flowers ranging from pure white to deep pink. Historically, water lilies were revered by ancient civilizations, notably the Egyptians, who associated them with creation and rebirth. Throughout the ages, water lily roots have been used for their medicinal properties. In traditional medicine, water lily has been used to treat a variety of conditions, such as gastrointestinal disorders, skin inflammations and sleep disorders. Asian cultures also attribute spiritual properties to the water lily, regarding it as a symbol of enlightenment and spiritual awakening.

In the kitchen

The water lily is not only an ornamental plant, it also has a place in the kitchen. Water lily seeds, known as **water nuts**, are particularly **nutritious** and can be eaten raw or cooked. They are **rich in starch** and can be used as a potato substitute. Young leaves and petals can be used in salads, adding a unique touch and delicate fragrance to your dishes. The rhizomes, meanwhile, are **rich in vitamins and minerals**, and can be cooked in a variety of ways, including in soups or purees. Water lilies are not only a delight to the eye, but also a treasure trove of **nutritional benefits**. Their use in cooking allows you to benefit from their **antioxidant** and **anti-inflammatory properties**, while adding an original and tasty touch to your recipes. However, it is crucial to ensure that the water lilies used are edible and not treated with chemicals, as not all species are edible and some may be toxic. By observing these precautions, water lilies can become a valuable and surprising addition to your kitchen, combining novel flavors and health benefits.

HEALING WITH WATER LILIES

- To soothe **insomnia**, infuse a handful of water-lily petals in a cup of boiling water for 10 minutes. Drink this tea before going to bed.

- If you have **skin problems,** apply a water-lily root poultice. Crush the roots into a paste and apply to the skin for 20 minutes.

- For **gastrointestinal irritations,** drink a decoction of water-lily roots. Boil a small quantity of roots in water and drink after each meal.

- For **diarrhea,** mix a teaspoon of dried water lily root in a glass of water and drink two or three times a day.

- For **kidney disorders,** use water lily as a natural diuretic. Drink water lily tea regularly.

- For **minor wounds** or cuts, apply fresh water lily juice directly to the wound, to help it heal.

WATER LILIES IN THE KITCHEN

Water Lily Petal Salad

INGREDIENTS: Water lily petals, 200g salad greens, 1 avocado, 100g walnuts, 1 tbsp balsamic vinegar, 3 tbsp olive oil, salt, pepper.

1. Gently wash the water lily petals and lettuce shoots.

2. Peel and slice the avocado.

3. Mix the petals, baby greens, avocado and walnuts in a large bowl.

4. In a small bowl, combine the balsamic vinegar, olive oil, salt and pepper to make a vinaigrette.

5. Pour the vinaigrette over the salad and toss gently.

6. Serve immediately and enjoy this refreshing, nutritious salad!

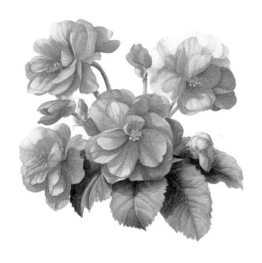

THE BEGONIA
(BEGONIA)

COMESTIBLE AND CURATIVE RADIANCE

The begonia, a well-known ornamental plant, dazzles us with its diversity of shapes and colors, but that's not all. In addition to its aesthetic appeal, it has astonishing culinary and medicinal properties.

Known primarily for its ornamental beauty, the begonia, native to tropical and subtropical regions, hides culinary and medicinal secrets. For centuries, different cultures have used this bright flower not only to decorate their gardens, but also in the preparation of natural remedies. Begonia flowers, stems and leaves are edible and appreciated for their lemony taste and crunchy texture. Central American natives used begonia to treat skin infections and sore throats. In Asia, begonia was used as a remedy for ulcers and as a liver tonic. This delicate plant is thus an unexpected source of health benefits, combining aesthetic, culinary and therapeutic qualities.

In the kitchen

Begonia offers an **explosion of flavors and textures** in the kitchen. Its petals can be used to **add a tangy touch** to salads or desserts. The stems and leaves, meanwhile, are often added to soups or sautéed with other vegetables. Begonia's **high vitamin C content** makes it an excellent antioxidant, and its ability to **reduce inflammation** makes it beneficial for digestive health. It is also considered **a natural remedy for skin infections and ulcers**. Begonias are also used to create refreshing drinks and medicinal teas, exploiting their diuretic and detoxifying properties. Begonias' antioxidant and anti-inflammatory properties are particularly valued in dishes, not only adding unique flavor but also health benefits. However, it's essential to know which variety of begonia to use in cooking, as some can be toxic. Their culinary use is therefore as delicate as their appearance, requiring special care and a thorough knowledge of their properties.

HEALING WITH BEGONIA

- For **skin inflammations**, crush fresh Begonia leaves and apply directly to the skin.

- To **soothe sore throats**, prepare an infusion of begonia leaves. Drink it two or three times a day.

- If you have **digestive problems,** eat raw begonia leaves in salads, as they have a calming effect on the digestive system.

- For **ulcers,** chew begonia leaves directly several times a day.

- To **combat urinary tract infections**, make a decoction with begonia stems and drink regularly.

- If you're suffering from **fatigue**, begonia tea can help revitalize the body and improve energy.

BEGONIA IN THE KITCHEN

Fresh Begonia Salad

INGREDIENTS: A few begonia leaves, 1 cucumber, 2 tomatoes, 1 avocado, 1 tablespoon balsamic vinegar, 2 tablespoons olive oil, salt and pepper.

1. Wash and chop the begonia leaves.
2. Peel and dice the cucumber, tomatoes and avocado.
3. Gently mix all the ingredients in a bowl.
4. Season with balsamic vinegar, olive oil, salt and pepper to taste.

5. Refrigerate for half an hour before serving. Enjoy this fresh, tangy salad with all its health benefits!

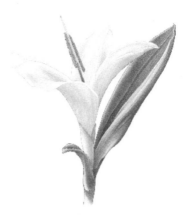

BANANA FLOWER
(MUSA)

A TROPICAL CULINARY TREASURE TROVE

Let's stop off in the tropics and subtropics to discover the banana flower, a culinary and medicinal marvel that adds an exotic touch to a variety of traditional dishes.

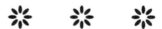

Banana flower, also known as "banana heart", is an edible flower that grows at the end of banana bunches in tropical regions. It is widely consumed in Southeast Asia, India and other tropical regions of the world. It is valued not only for its nutritional and medicinal benefits, but also for its delicate texture and unique taste. Used for centuries in traditional medicine for its anti-inflammatory and antioxidant properties, banana blossom is rich in vitamins A and C, fiber and essential minerals such as potassium and magnesium. Ayurvedic medicine also attributes beneficial properties to improve digestion and treat infections. Historically, in many cultures, it has been used to improve women's reproductive and menstrual health, and is considered a therapeutic food in many culinary traditions. Banana blossom is a low-calorie food that contributes to a healthy, balanced diet.

In the kitchen

Banana flower is a versatile ingredient that can be transformed into a variety of delicious dishes, from salads to curries. It is best known for **improving digestion** and **reducing inflammation**. Chefs appreciate its tender texture and slightly bitter taste, and use it in salads, soups and stir-fry dishes. Its **anti-inflammatory** and **antioxidant properties make it a** healthy addition to any diet. Banana blossom can be eaten raw, steamed, fried or boiled, and can be added to a multitude of traditional recipes, giving it a unique and exotic flavor. An important aspect to consider when cooking banana blossom is its pre-treatment, which usually involves removing the hard outer bracts and buds, and soaking the blossom in acidulated water to prevent oxidation. Proper preparation of banana flower reveals a nutritious and delicious food that can enhance many culinary preparations, enriching dishes with its health-giving qualities. However, it should be eaten in moderation due to its tannin content, which can cause stomach upsets in some people.

HEALING WITH BANANA BLOSSOM

- To **improve digestion**, make a decoction from banana blossoms. Cut a banana flower into pieces and boil in water for 15 minutes. Strain and drink once a day.

- For **painful menstruation,** eat banana blossom as a salad or cooked dish to ease the pain.

- To **reduce inflammation,** include banana blossoms in your diet on a regular basis.

- If you have **diabetes,** include banana blossom in your diet to regulate blood glucose levels.

- For **anemia,** eat dishes cooked with banana blossom to increase hemoglobin levels in the blood.

- For **lactation problems**, use banana flower in salads or dishes to improve milk production in nursing mothers.

BANANA FLOWER IN THE KITCHEN

Banana Flower Salad

INGREDIENTS: 1 banana flower, 2 tbsp lemon juice, 1 cup shredded coconut, 2 chopped green chillies, salt to taste, fresh coriander to garnish.

1. Prepare the banana flower by removing the outer bracts and thinly slicing the edible part. Soak in lemon water to prevent oxidation.

2. Mix sliced banana flower with lemon juice, salt, green chillies and shredded coconut.

3. Garnish with fresh coriander and serve immediately as a refreshing and nutritious side dish. Enjoy this exotic salad full of flavor and health benefits!

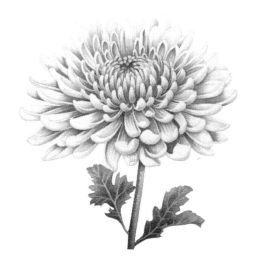

THE CHRYSANTHEMUM
(CHRYSANTHEMUM)

AN ELIXIR OF LONGEVITY

Let's take a tour of Asia's flourishing paths to discover a flower with many virtues, the Chrysanthemum, a symbol of longevity and harmonious life.

Native to China, the Chrysanthemum is a magnificent flower, appreciated for its beauty and multiple benefits since ancient times. This perennial plant, which blooms in autumn, is symbolic of longevity and health. The Chinese have been cultivating it since the 15th century BC, and have incorporated it into various aspects of their lives, including traditional medicine and gastronomy. Chrysanthemum infusions are renowned for their ability to clear the eyes and improve eyesight, soothe the mind, and increase longevity. They are also appreciated for their anti-inflammatory, anti-aging and antipyretic properties. The Japanese, in awe of this flower, have even dedicated the National Chrysanthemum Festival to celebrating its virtues. The Chrysanthemum then spread throughout the world, enriching various cultures with its benefits and beauty, while becoming a popular ornamental flower.

In the kitchen

Chrysanthemums are used in a variety of cuisines, particularly in Asia. **Infused**, it makes a floral, refreshing and aromatic drink. Young, tender Chrysanthemum leaves are also **eaten in salads** or **sautéed** as a green vegetable. Rich in **vitamins A and C**, Chrysanthemum is an ally for **eye and skin health,** and a **powerful antioxidant**. Its **anti-inflammatory properties** help combat various inflammations and infections. Chrysanthemum infusion is also known to **relax the nerves** and contribute to good **cardiovascular health**. It is often incorporated into sweet and savory dishes for its floral touches, offering a unique and delicate flavor dimension. Its **distinctive flavor makes it an** ingredient of choice for many traditional and modern recipes, creating an explosion of flavors and benefits for those who enjoy it. Be careful, however, about the origin of chrysanthemum flowers used in cooking: they must be free from pesticides and other chemicals, so choose food-grade flowers.

TAKING CARE OF YOURSELF WITH CHRYSANTHEMUMS

- To **soothe tired eyes**, infuse dried chrysanthemum flowers in hot water and use as an eye lotion.

- In case of **headache** or **fever,** drink an infusion of chrysanthemum several times a day.
  - To **improve digestion** and treat **constipation**, drink chrysanthemum tea regularly.

- If you have **skin problems** such as acne, apply a compress of infused chrysanthemum flowers to the affected areas.

- To relieve **cold symptoms,** prepare an infusion of chrysanthemum mixed with fresh ginger.

- For **insomnia,** drink a cup of chrysanthemum tea before going to bed.

- If you suffer from **high blood pressure,** make chrysanthemum tea a regular part of your diet.

CHRYSANTHEMUMS IN THE KITCHEN

Chrysanthemum Salad

INGREDIENTS: 1 cup young chrysanthemum leaves, 2 tbsp olive oil, 1 tbsp rice vinegar, 1 tsp honey, salt and pepper to taste, 1 tbsp toasted sesame seeds.

1. Wash young chrysanthemum leaves and spin dry.

2. In a bowl, mix olive oil, rice vinegar, honey, salt and pepper to create a vinaigrette.

3. Pour the vinaigrette over the chrysanthemum leaves and toss well to coat.

4. Sprinkle with toasted sesame seeds before serving. This salad can be served as a refreshing and tasty starter.

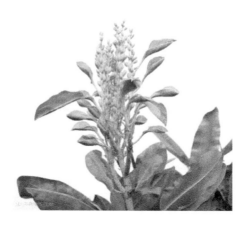

THE COCONUT FLOWER
(COCOS NUCIFERA)

A TROPICAL ELIXIR

Let's dive into the heart of tropical regions to discover a hidden treasure: the coconut flower. Less well known than its fruit, the coconut, this flower is an exceptional ingredient with multiple virtues.

The coconut palm is a member of the Arecaceae family and is widely distributed in tropical and subtropical regions of the world. This versatile plant has been honored and used for centuries by local communities. Ancient Ayurvedic and Siddha texts cite coconut flower for its nutritional and medicinal benefits. Coconut blossom sap is traditionally harvested to produce coconut sugar, a natural sweetener, and palm wine. It is a symbol of prosperity and fertility in many cultures and religions, often associated with life and immortality. The coconut flower, with its creamy shades and soft petals, is a rich source of nutrients, such as vitamins, minerals and antioxidants. Its medicinal uses include the treatment of kidney disease, hypertension and diabetes. Ancient cultures value coconut blossom for its antibacterial, anti-inflammatory and antiviral properties, as well as for its potential to improve digestion and strengthen the immune system.

In the kitchen

Coconut blossom is an exotic ingredient that **enhances the flavour of** sweet and savoury dishes. In particular, **coconut flower nectar** is a natural, healthy sweetener and alternative to white sugar, offering a sweet, caramelized taste. It is **rich in vitamins and minerals, and** is an **excellent sugar substitute for** diabetics. Coconut sugar, derived from the sap of the coconut blossom, is not only nutritious, but also environmentally friendly, making it a sustainable choice. Coconut blossoms, with their intrinsic sweetness, are also used in various Asian cuisines to concoct tasty dishes and desserts. **Coconut blossom sap** can be fermented to produce coconut vinegar and palm wine, two products valued for their probiotic properties beneficial to **intestinal health**. It is also the basis of many traditional and medicinal dishes in various parts of the world. Coconut blossom's **antioxidant** and **anti-inflammatory** properties are not only beneficial to health, but also add a nutritious dimension to dishes. Amateur and professional chefs alike exploit the flower essence to enrich their culinary creations, from starters to desserts and drinks, adding a unique tropical touch to their recipes.

HEALING WITH COCONUT FLOWER

- **For hypertension and diabetes**, regular consumption of coconut flower sap can help. Mix a tablespoon of sap in a glass of water and drink the mixture every morning.

- For **kidney problems**, prepare a decoction by boiling one tablespoon of dried flowers in two cups of water until reduced by half. Drink this decoction twice a day.

- **To boost the immune system**, mix coconut flower nectar with hot water and drink this solution regularly.

- **Skin problems and inflammation** can be treated by applying a local poultice of crushed coconut flowers.

- For **digestive problems,** consume coconut sugar regularly, as it is a natural probiotic.

- **For mouth infections,** rinse mouth with coconut flower-infused water several times a day.

- In the case of **inflammatory diseases,** regular incorporation of coconut blossoms into the diet can offer relief.

COCONUT FLOWER IN THE KITCHEN

Coconut flower rice

INGREDIENTS: 200 g basmati rice, 100 g fresh coconut flowers, 1 tbsp coconut oil, 1 tsp salt, 400 ml water.

1. Rinse the rice until the water runs clear.

2. Heat the coconut oil in a saucepan and add the coconut blossoms. Sauté until tender.

3. Add the rice and sauté with the flowers until well coated with oil.

4. Add water and salt, bring to the boil, then reduce heat and cover. Cook for 18 minutes.

5. Turn off the heat and leave the rice to rest for 5 minutes before serving. Enjoy this exotic dish with its subtle flavours and the benefits of coconut blossom!

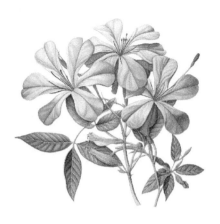

PLUMBAGO
(PLUMBAGO AURICULATA)

A JOURNEY OF BENEFITS

Decorative and medicinal, plumbago is a versatile plant, combining beauty and utility, from tropical and subtropical regions.

Native to South Africa, plumbago, also known as "lacewort", is an ornamental and medicinal plant with blue or white flowers. Plumbago's diverse uses have spanned the ages and continents. In traditional medicine, it is renowned for its anti-inflammatory and analgesic properties, used to treat various skin conditions and digestive disorders. Plumbago was also used by some ancient cultures as a remedy for snakebites and infections. Its leaves and roots are used in traditional Indian medicine (Ayurveda) to treat skin diseases, boils and sore throats. This plant has gained worldwide recognition not only for its beauty as an ornamental plant, but also for its role in traditional medicine.

In the kitchen

Plumbago, although primarily an ornamental and medicinal plant, also finds a place in some kitchens, especially for its **medicinal properties**. Its leaves, often used in infusions, are known to **soothe sore throats** and **relieve digestive disorders**. It is not commonly used in everyday cooking due to its potent active compounds, and its use should be approached with caution. However, it is sometimes incorporated into traditional dishes to **boost immunity** and fight infection. Plumbago leaves, when added in moderate quantities to herbal teas or soups, can **boost the** body's **natural defenses, combat inflammation** and provide **relief from joint pain**. Used judiciously, this plant can offer numerous health benefits. However, the culinary use of plumbago must be done with discernment due to its potentially strong effects, and it is crucial to respect the recommended dosages to avoid any undesirable side effects.

TREATING YOURSELF WITH PLUMBAGO

- To **soothe skin pain**, apply a paste made from crushed plumbago leaves to the affected area.

- For **digestive problems**, prepare an infusion with a teaspoon of dried plumbago root in a cup of boiling water and drink.

- For **skin inflammations and infections**, apply the juice extracted from plumbago leaves directly to the skin.

- For **sore throats,** gargle with an infusion of plumbago leaves.

- In the case of **snakebite,** a paste of plumbago root applied to the bite can help.

- For **immune disorders,** regular consumption of small quantities of plumbago can boost the immune system.

- For **respiratory problems,** inhale a steam decoction of plumbago leaves.

PLUMBAGO IN THE KITCHEN

Soothing Plumbago Herbal Tea

INGREDIENTS: 1 tsp dried plumbago leaves, 1 cup water, Honey (optional), Lemon (optional).

1. Bring the water to the boil.
2. Add the dried plumbago leaves to the boiling water.
3. Cover and leave to infuse for 5 to 10 minutes.

4. Strain the leaves and pour the tea into a cup.

5. Add honey or lemon to taste, if desired.

6. Enjoy the herbal tea while taking advantage of its health-giving properties.

Remember that plumbago is powerful and should be used with caution and in moderate quantities. Always consult a health care professional before starting any herbal treatment, especially if you are pregnant, breastfeeding, have existing medical conditions or are taking medication.

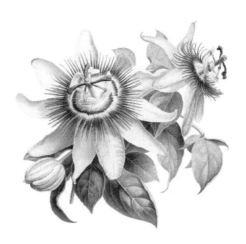

THE PASSIFLORA
(PASSIFLORA)

TROPICAL CALM AND TRANQUILLITY

Let's embark on an exotic journey to the tropical and subtropical regions of South America to discover passionflower, the intriguing and spectacular flower also known as passion flower.

Native to the tropical and subtropical regions of South America, passionflower is renowned for its unique beauty and medicinal properties. The Spaniards discovered it in the 16th century and were fascinated by its flower, which they thought symbolized the Passion of Christ, hence its name. This perennial liana is grown all over the world for its flowers, fruit and therapeutic virtues. In traditional medicine, passionflower has been used to treat a variety of ailments, from insomnia and anxiety to inflammations and burns. It is a well-known remedy for **calming the nerves** and **promoting sleep**. Passionflower is also rich in vitamins, minerals and antioxidants, making it an excellent supplement for promoting optimal health.

In the kitchen

Passionflower, best known as passion fruit, is an **exotic** and **versatile** ingredient. It is **rich in vitamins A and C**, **fiber** and **antioxidants** that are essential for human health. The fruit is often eaten fresh, but is also delicious in drinks, salads, desserts and sauces. Passion fruit's unique sweet-tart taste can enhance many dishes and beverages. A passionflower syrup can be made to flavor cocktails or desserts. In addition, passionflower leaves can be used to make soothing herbal teas, perfect for **relaxing** the mind and body after a stressful day. Passionflower flowers can also be used to make a soothing infusion, often used to combat insomnia. Although less well-known for its use in cooking, passionflower is an incredible source of flavor and health benefits, adding a tropical touch and a twist to dishes.

TAKING CARE OF YOURSELF WITH PASSIONFLOWER

- To combat **insomnia**, infuse a tablespoon of dried passionflowers in a cup of boiling water for 10 minutes. Drink this infusion before going to bed.

- In case of **stress** or **anxiety,** mix a few drops of passionflower extract in water or a drink and consume as needed.

- For **burns** or skin irritations, apply a passionflower-based ointment directly to the affected area several times a day.

- For **skin infections** or **acne**, apply a few drops of passionflower essential oil diluted in a vegetable oil to the affected areas.

- If you suffer from **muscular tension** or **headaches**, infuse passionflower leaves in hot water and drink as an herbal tea.

- For **digestive disorders,** drink passionflower tea regularly to soothe the digestive system.

- In case of **hypertension,** consume passionflower extract regularly under medical supervision.

PASSIONFLOWER IN THE KITCHEN

Passionflower Sorbet

INGREDIENTS: 500 ml passion fruit pulp, 200 g sugar, 250 ml water, juice of one lemon.

1. Mix the water and sugar in a saucepan and bring to the boil to make a syrup. Leave to cool.

2. Mix the passion fruit pulp with the lemon juice and cooled syrup.

3. Strain the mixture through a sieve to remove the seeds.

4. Pour the mixture into an ice-cream maker and whirl until firm.

5. Place the sorbet in the freezer until set. Serve chilled and enjoy!

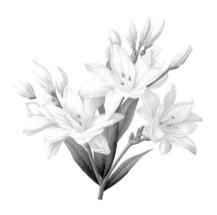

THE TUBERUSE
(POLIANTHES TUBEROSA)

BEWITCHING FRAGRANCE AND NOCTURNAL CHARM

Let's embark on an olfactory journey into the enchanting world of tuberose, a flower whose intense, bewitching fragrance reveals itself at dusk, evoking mystery and fascination.

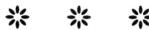

Native to Mexico, tuberose, with its powerful, voluptuous fragrance, has captivated hearts since ancient times. Its white flowers, renowned for their intoxicating aroma, bloom at nightfall. In ancient Mesopotamia, it symbolized protection and harmony. Transported to

Europe in the 17th century, it quickly became a centerpiece of royal gardens and perfume compositions. Tuberose is distinguished not only by its aroma, but also by its representation of sensuality and passion in different cultures. It is often associated with forbidden feelings and deep desires. In perfumery, it remains a precious ingredient, appreciated for its warm, exotic note. The fragrance of tuberose is complex, blending nuances of honey, banana and spice, all on a creamy, velvety base.

In the kitchen

Tuberose offers a unique, captivating floral note that can transcend a variety of culinary preparations. Its **exotic, sensual aroma** blends perfectly with creamy desserts and beverages. Tuberose petals, infused in syrups or creams, add a delicate, bewitching touch. **As an infusion,** it gives off sweet and spicy nuances, adding a sophisticated dimension to cocktails and hot drinks. Although less common in cooking than other edible flowers, tuberose deserves a place of honor in modern gastronomy for its delicate, inimitable fragrance. Used sparingly, it can transform an ordinary recipe into a sublime dish, seducing palates with its voluptuous, intoxicating floral notes. Chefs and lovers of experimental cuisine find tuberose an inexhaustible source of inspiration for creating dishes that are a true tribute to the aromatic richness of this majestic flower. Ultimately, tuberose, with its unique aromatic properties, enriches the culinary arts by adding a touch of mystery and sophistication to every dish.

HEALING WITH TUBEROSE

- To soothe **stress** and **anxiety**, take a few dried tuberose petals and steep them in hot water. Inhale deeply to calm the mind.

- For **skin problems**, infuse tuberose petals in sweet almond oil. Apply this infused oil to the skin to nourish and moisturize.

- If you're feeling **tense,** diffuse tuberose essential oil in your environment. Its relaxing fragrance helps reduce tension.

- For a good **night's sleep,** place tuberose petals under your pillow. The enchanting aroma promotes peaceful sleep.

- For **dry skin**, create an oil bath by mixing tuberose petals with a base oil. Apply to skin to rehydrate.

- In case of **melancholy** or **depression,** inhale tuberose aroma regularly. Its comforting fragrance soothes the mind and balances emotions.

TUBEROSE IN THE KITCHEN

Crème Brûlée with Tuberose

INGREDIENTS: 500 ml liquid cream, 1 vanilla pod, 5 egg yolks, 100 g sugar, a few dried tuberose petals.

- Preheat oven to 150°C.

- Heat the cream with the split vanilla pod and tuberose petals. Leave to infuse.

- Whisk the egg yolks with the sugar until the mixture whitens.

- Remove the vanilla pod from the cream and pour over the egg and sugar mixture, stirring constantly.

- Strain the mixture and pour into ramekins.

- Place the ramekins in a bain-marie and bake for 35 minutes.

- Once cooled, sprinkle with sugar and caramelize with a kitchen blowtorch. Enjoy this tuberose-flavored crème brûlée!

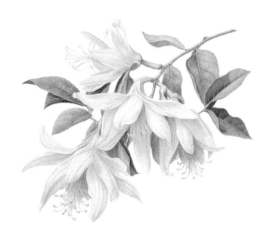

YLANG-YLANG
(CANANGA ODORATA)

FOR EXQUISITE SENSUALITY

Discover Ylang-Ylang, an exotic flower renowned for its sweet, bewitching fragrance, highly prized in perfumery, but which is also used in the culinary arts and has exceptional therapeutic virtues.

Ylang-Ylang, native to Indonesia and Madagascar, is a precious, fragrant flower of the Cananga odorata tree. This bright yellow flower is often associated with romance and relaxation. For centuries, it has been used in beauty rituals and wellness treatments for its soothing and revitalizing properties. In the Pacific islands, Ylang-Ylang oil has traditionally been used to concoct aromatic preparations and massage oils for its relaxing effect and sensual aroma. Ylang-Ylang's therapeutic qualities and bewitching fragrance make it a choice ingredient in luxury perfumery and high-end cosmetics. Its essence made its way to Europe in the 19th century, where it quickly seduced the finest noses. In addition to its relaxing properties, Ylang-Ylang is also said to be a natural aphrodisiac, and is used in various ways in cultures around the world to uplift the spirit and soothe body and soul.

In the kitchen

Ylang-Ylang is also a treasure in the kitchen, especially for delicately perfuming desserts and drinks. In particular, its unique aroma **enriches** sweet preparations, giving them an exquisite floral note. Its **antioxidant** and **anti-inflammatory** properties offer not only health benefits but also an inimitable taste. A few drops of Ylang-Ylang essential oil can transform a simple dish into an exceptional gastronomic experience, revealing subtle and original flavors. In addition to its gustatory virtues, Ylang-Ylang is also prized for its benefits on well-being and mental health, helping to **reduce stress and anxiety**, and promoting a sense of **peace** and **relaxation**. It's an ideal ingredient for dishes intended for a romantic dinner or a moment of relaxation. The blossoming of Ylang-Ylang offers not only an explosion of flavors in the kitchen, but also an invitation to travel, to discover new sensations and a world of relaxation and pleasure. So don't hesitate to experiment with this enchanting flower to elevate your culinary preparations to a new level of delectation and finesse.

TREATING YOURSELF WITH YLANG-YLANG

- To relieve **stress and anxiety**, place a few drops of Ylang-Ylang essential oil in a diffuser or inhale directly from the bottle.

- For **skin problems** such as acne, mix a few drops of Ylang-Ylang essential oil with a carrier oil and apply to the skin.

- For **insomnia and sleep disorders**, add a few drops of Ylang-Ylang essential oil to your bath before bedtime.

- For **high blood pressure,** mix a few drops of Ylang-Ylang essential oil with a vegetable oil and gently massage the body.

- If you have **hair or scalp problems,** add a few drops of Ylang-Ylang essential oil to your usual shampoo or conditioner.

- To treat **mild to moderate depression**, inhale the aroma of Ylang-Ylang regularly or use an essential oil diffuser in your living space.

YLANG-YLANG IN THE KITCHEN

Ylang-Ylang Sorbet

INGREDIENTS: 500 ml water, 200 g sugar, 2 tbsp Ylang-Ylang syrup, juice of 2 lemons.

1. Bring water and sugar to the boil until syrupy.

2. Remove from the heat and add the Ylang-Ylang syrup and lemon juice. Mix well.

3. Allow the mixture to cool, then pour into a freezer-safe container.

4. Set the sorbet in the freezer, stirring occasionally to prevent ice crystals from forming.

5. Once the sorbet has set, serve it in balls in bowls. Enjoy this fragrant, exotic delight!

PART III: WILD NORTH AMERICAN EDIBLE FLOWERS

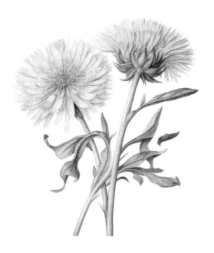

LION'S-TOOTH
(TARAXACUM OFFICINALE)

For flourishing health

Let's delve into the fascinating world of edible flowers, where the Lion's Tooth, often considered a mere weed, reigns supreme thanks to its many health benefits.

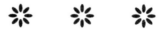

Lion's-tooth, is a ubiquitous wildflower in meadows and gardens the world over. Recognizable by its serrated leaves and bright yellow flowers, this plant has a long history of both culinary and medicinal use. Since ancient times, various cultures have valued Lion's Tooth for its diverse medicinal properties, such as its diuretic and detoxifying effects. In traditional Chinese medicine, it is used to strengthen the liver, eliminate heat and resolve toxicity. In traditional European medicine, Lion's Tooth has been valued for treating digestive disorders, inflammation and infections. Its leaves, flowers and roots are used to concoct herbal teas, salads, medicinal vinegars and even wine.

In the kitchen

Lion's Tooth is a treasure trove of **nutritional goodness**, packed with vitamins A, C and K, as well as calcium, potassium and iron. **Rich in antioxidants**, its leaves add a bitter, tangy note to salads and can be sautéed like spinach. The flowers, with their milder taste, can decorate dishes or be made into syrup. The roots, meanwhile, can be roasted to make a coffee-like beverage. As well as being **nourishing and detoxifying**, Lion's Tooth has **diuretic properties** that make it beneficial for the liver and kidneys, helping to eliminate toxins from the body. In the kitchen, Lion's Tooth is versatile, enhancing a variety of dishes with its unique flavor, adding an **earthy, bitter note** that contrasts nicely with milder ingredients. Dent-de-Lion is therefore a welcome addition to healthy, gourmet cooking, bringing a balance of flavors and a myriad of **health benefits**.

HEALING WITH LION'S TEETH

- For **water retention**, make an herbal tea by infusing a tablespoon of dried Lion's Tooth leaves in boiling water for 10 minutes. Drink three times a day.

- For **digestive problems**, eat raw young Lion's Tooth leaves in salads to aid digestion and for their diuretic effects.

- For a **sore throat**, make a herbal tea with Dent-de-Lion flowers, a tablespoon of honey and a slice of lemon. Leave to infuse for 10 minutes and drink hot.

- For **liver disorders**, prepare a decoction of Lion's Tooth root and drink one cup before each meal.

- For **acne,** apply Lion's Tooth stem juice directly to pimples for its antibacterial and anti-inflammatory properties.

- For **fatigue,** mix fresh Lion's Tooth juice with lemon juice and honey as a tonic.

- If you suffer from **constipation,** the fiber-rich Lion's Tooth can help regulate intestinal transit when eaten regularly in salads.

LION'S-TOOTH IN THE KITCHEN

Lion's-tooth salad with bacon

INGREDIENTS: A handful of young Lion's-tooth leaves, 100 g bacon, 1 shallot, 1 tablespoon cider vinegar, 2 tablespoons olive oil, salt, pepper.

1. Wash and drain the Lion's-tooth leaves well.

2. Fry the lardons in a fat-free frying pan until golden and crisp.

3. Thinly slice the shallot and add it to the lardons, then sauté for a few minutes.

4. Deglaze the pan with the cider vinegar and add the olive oil.

5. Pour over the Lion's-tooth leaves.

6. Mix well, season to taste, and serve immediately. Enjoy your meal!

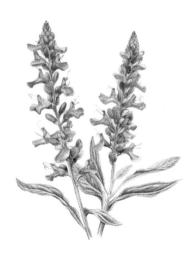

MEADOW SAGE
(SALVIA PRATENSIS)

A NATURAL REMEDY

Roam the fields and meadows of Europe to discover a herb with many virtues: Meadow Sage, used both for its medicinal properties and its aroma in cooking.

Meadow Sage, or Salvia pratensis, is a hardy perennial that thrives in the meadows of Europe and Western Asia. With its violet flowers and distinctive fragrance, this plant has been used through the ages for its medicinal and culinary properties. The Greeks and Romans used it to improve memory and protect against various ailments. In the Middle Ages, it was cultivated in monastic gardens for its digestive, anti-inflammatory and antiseptic virtues. Meadow Sage has also played an important role in folk medicine to treat throat disorders, coughs, mouth inflammations and toothache. It has also been used to improve digestion and treat menstrual disorders and excessive perspiration. Meadow Sage, with its wealth of bioactive compounds, continues to be a mainstay of modern phytotherapy.

In the kitchen

Meadow Sage, with its aromatic, earthy fragrance, **enhances meat dishes**, sauces and pasta dishes. It blends well with garlic, lemon and olive oil, adding a deep, complex flavor. **Antiseptic and digestive**, it is often used in infusions to relieve various gastrointestinal disorders. Used fresh or dried, it retains most of its **aromatic** and **medicinal properties**. Adding sage to your dishes can **aid digestion** and add an unexpected layer of flavor. However, use in moderation, as its dominant flavor can overwhelm other ingredients. Meadow Sage offers an interesting alternative to common sage in cooking, bringing a unique nuance and a wealth of health benefits. In short, incorporating this herb into your recipes can not only **enhance the flavor of your dishes, but** also **take advantage of its many health benefits**. For those looking to expand their culinary repertoire while incorporating healthy foods, Meadow Sage is a great place to start.

TAKING CARE OF YOURSELF WITH MEADOW SAGE

- For **digestive problems**, infuse a teaspoon of meadow sage leaves in a cup of boiling water for 10 minutes. Strain and drink after meals.

- For **sore throats,** gargle with an infusion of meadow sage mixed with salt.

- For **skin infections**, apply a compress soaked in meadow sage infusion to the affected area.

- For **excessive perspiration,** drink an infusion of meadow sage regularly.

- To relieve **premenstrual symptoms,** infuse meadow sage leaves and drink the infusion twice a day.

- If you have **gum problems,** use a decoction of meadow sage as a mouthwash.

- For **coughs and headaches,** inhale the vapors from an infusion of meadow sage.

MEADOW SAGE IN THE KITCHEN

Pasta with Meadow Sage

INGREDIENTS: 300 g pasta, 2 tbsp olive oil, 1 tsp chopped meadow sage leaves, salt, pepper, 50 g grated Parmesan cheese.

1. Cook pasta according to package instructions.

2. Meanwhile, heat the olive oil in a frying pan and sauté the chopped meadow sage for 1-2 minutes.

3. Drain the pasta and add it to the pan with the meadow sage. Mix well to coat the pasta.

4. Season with salt and pepper to taste and sprinkle with grated Parmesan before serving. Enjoy and discover the unique flavor of meadow sage!

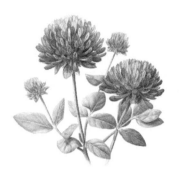

RED CLOVER
(TRIFOLIUM PRATENSE)

A BOTANICAL TREASURE WITH MULTIPLE BENEFITS

Enrich your knowledge of plants by discovering red clover, a remarkable plant with multiple therapeutic properties, native to Europe, North Africa and Western Asia.

Red clover is a well-known perennial plant, recognizable by its red flowers and trifoliate leaves. It has been valued throughout history for its medicinal and nutritional benefits. Traditionally used by various cultures, red clover was notably used to treat skin ailments, coughs and menopausal conditions. Native Americans used it to soothe muscle cramps and as a tonic to purify the blood. In China, it was prized for its detoxifying and anti-inflammatory properties. Red clover is rich in isoflavones, phytochemical compounds with antioxidant and estrogenic effects. These compounds give it beneficial properties against menopausal disorders, osteoporosis and cardiovascular disease. In addition, red clover leaves are rich in vitamins and minerals, making it an ideal nutritional supplement. Today, it is widely used in herbal teas, dietary supplements and tinctures, and continues to play an important role in both traditional and modern medicine.

In the kitchen

Red clover is not only valued for its medicinal properties; it also occupies an interesting place in the kitchen. The young leaves and flowers of red clover are **edible** and can be added to salads for a touch of color and delicate flavor. The flowers have a sweet taste and are often used to make syrups and jams. Red clover is also **rich in protein**, making it particularly nutritious. The leaves, once dried, can be used as a **tea substitute**, providing a sweet, soothing drink, rich in **antioxidants** and beneficial for **cardiovascular health**. Incorporating red clover into your diet can be an enjoyable and nutritious way to enjoy its many **health benefits**. Whether as a garnish, an infusion or a delicious syrup, red clover is a versatile and healthy addition to everyday cooking. Beware, however, of consuming red clover in moderation, especially for people with blood coagulation disorders, due to its coumarin content, a natural anticoagulant.

HEALING WITH RED CLOVER

- In case of **cough** or **congestion**, prepare a herbal tea by infusing a tablespoon of red clover flowers in a cup of boiling water for 5 to 10 minutes. Drink up to three times a day.

- For **skin infections** or **inflammation**, apply a paste made from crushed red clover flowers directly to the affected area.

- If you are suffering from **menopausal disorders**, consume red clover regularly as an herbal tea or dietary supplement, after consulting a health professional.

- For **digestive problems,** take red clover tea before meals to stimulate digestion.

- For **eczema** or **skin irritation**, apply a red clover-based cream to the affected area twice a day.

- To boost the **immune system**, consume red clover regularly as an herbal tea or supplement.

- To combat **water retention**, red clover acts as a natural diuretic. Use it as an herbal tea to benefit from this effect.

RED CLOVER IN THE KITCHEN

Red Clover Salad

INGREDIENTS: A handful of red clover flowers, 200 g lettuce, 1 sliced cucumber, 150 g halved cherry tomatoes, 50 g walnuts, 2 tbsp olive oil, 1 tbsp balsamic vinegar, salt, pepper.

1. Wash the red clover flowers and leave to dry.
2. In a large salad bowl, combine the lettuce, cucumber, cherry tomatoes and red clover blossoms.
3. In a small bowl, combine the olive oil, balsamic vinegar, salt and pepper to make a vinaigrette.
4. Pour the vinaigrette over the salad and toss well.
5. Garnish the salad with walnuts before serving.
6. Enjoy this delicious salad, rich in flavour and health benefits!

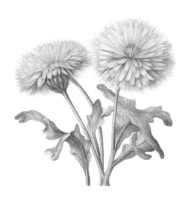

DANDELION
(TARAXACUM)

A HIDDEN GARDEN TREASURE

Let's delve into the fascinating world of wild plants with a humble and common herb: the dandelion, often considered a weed, but harboring many beneficial properties.

Dandelion, a common plant with bright yellow flowers, is well known to gardeners as an invasive weed. However, its reputation masks its important role in phytotherapy and its high nutritional value. Native to Eurasia, dandelion has been used since ancient times to treat a variety of ailments, including liver and digestive problems. The Greeks and Romans used it as a diuretic, while in the Middle Ages it was commonly used to treat liver and gall-bladder ailments, and as a remedy against infections. Native Americans also used dandelion to relieve digestive and skin disorders. With its deep roots, dandelion absorbs many minerals from the soil. Its leaves, flowers and roots are used to make medicines, teas, salads and even wines. Every part of this versatile plant is rich in nutrients, vitamins and minerals, and has **antioxidant**, **anti-inflammatory** and **diuretic** properties. Its leaves are an excellent dietary supplement, especially for those looking to add iron and calcium to their diet.

In the kitchen

Dandelion offers an abundance of flavor and nutrients in the kitchen. Its young leaves can be used raw in salads, adding a pleasantly bitter touch that **stimulates digestion** and **provides vitamins A and K**. More mature leaves can be cooked like spinach, adding depth of flavor and **rich mineral content**. The flowers, meanwhile, are often used to make syrups, jams or even dandelion wine, known for its **revitalizing** and **detoxifying** properties. Roasted and ground dandelion roots are a caffeine-free alternative to coffee, reputed to **stimulate digestion** and **support liver health**. **An antioxidant** and **diuretic,** dandelion is a valuable ally for those seeking to maintain a healthy lifestyle. It goes well with a variety of ingredients and can be incorporated into many dishes, adding a nutritious and therapeutic touch to your daily diet. Be careful, however, not to eat dandelions harvested by the roadside or in areas treated with pesticides.

TAKING CARE OF YOURSELF WITH DANDELION

- **For digestive disorders,** infuse a tablespoon of dried dandelion root in hot water for 10 minutes. Drink this tea two or three times a day.

- **For urinary tract infections or kidney problems**, prepare a decoction of fresh dandelion leaves and drink it throughout the day.

- **For water retention,** regularly eat salads of young dandelion leaves, which are an excellent natural diuretic.

- **For skin problems such as acne,** apply dandelion stem juice directly to the affected areas several times a day.

- **If you suffer from a sore throat,** gargle with an infusion of dandelion flowers mixed with honey to soothe an irritated throat.

- **For joint pain**, gently rub dandelion-infused oil over painful areas to relieve pain and inflammation.

- **To boost the immune system**, consume dandelion-infused honey regularly, as it's an excellent tonic.

DANDELION IN THE KITCHEN

Dandelion and Bacon Salad

INGREDIENTS: A handful of young dandelion leaves, 100 g bacon, 1 hard-boiled egg, 1 tbsp red wine vinegar, 2 tbsp olive oil, salt and pepper.

1. Wash and spin-dry young dandelion leaves.
2. Fry the lardons in a frying pan until crisp.
3. Mix the dandelion leaves, bacon and quartered hard-boiled egg in a bowl.
4. Prepare a vinaigrette with vinegar, olive oil, salt and pepper. Pour over salad and toss well.
5. Serve immediately and enjoy this delicious salad full of flavor and health benefits.

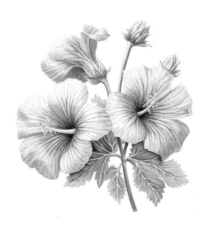

MALLOW
(MALVA)

A MEDICINAL SWEETNESS

Let's embark on a journey through the virtues of mallow, the purple and pink flower synonymous with sweetness and health benefits.

Legendary for its delicacy and beauty, mallow has been a prized medicinal plant in many cultures over the centuries. The Romans used it for its anti-inflammatory and soothing properties, adding it to their diet to treat sore throats and internal inflammation. The Egyptians used it to relieve skin irritations and respiratory problems. Mallow's history extends across Europe, Asia and North Africa, where it has been valued for its multiple benefits, such as relieving coughs, skin inflammations and even digestive problems. Mallow is recognized for its emollient, expectorant and anti-inflammatory properties, and is often incorporated into herbal remedies to treat various ailments and improve general health.

In the kitchen

Mallow can be a **beneficial and tasty addition to** a variety of dishes and recipes. **Rich in vitamins and minerals**, it can be used in salads to give a touch of color and a delicate taste or infused to take advantage of its **soothing and anti-inflammatory** benefits. Mallow flowers and leaves are **particularly useful for relieving gastrointestinal inflammation**, while the seeds can be used as a cheese substitute in certain vegetarian dishes. In addition, mallow's **emollient and moisturizing properties** make it ideal for concocting soups and sauces, providing not only a creamy texture, but also nutritional value. It is an excellent ingredient for those seeking to diversify their diet and incorporate essential nutrients in a delicate, tasty way. Be careful, however, to wash mallow thoroughly before eating to remove any residues or impurities, and to consume it in moderation, especially for those with a history of gastrointestinal disorders, to avoid any inconvenience.

HEALING WITH MALLOW

- To **relieve coughs and sore throats**, make an herbal tea with a teaspoon of dried mallow flowers and 250 ml of boiling water. Leave to infuse for 10 minutes, strain and drink up to 3 cups a day.

- For **skin inflammations**, apply a compress of infused mallow flowers to the affected area several times a day.

- For **digestive problems**, drink an infusion of mallow (15 g of flowers per 1 liter of water) to soothe inflammation and promote digestion.

- If you suffer from **constipation,** mallow, rich in mucilage, can act as a mild laxative. Use regularly as a herbal tea.

- For **respiratory tract irritation,** steam inhalation of a decoction of mallow flowers can be beneficial.

- For **acne and other skin blemishes**, apply a paste of crushed mallow flowers mixed with a little water, as a mask on the face.

MALLOW IN THE KITCHEN

Mallow salad

INGREDIENTS: 1 handful fresh mallow flowers, 200 g baby spinach, 1 avocado, 1 tablespoon olive oil, 1 tablespoon balsamic vinegar, salt and pepper.

1. Wash and drain the mallow flowers and baby spinach.

2. Peel and thinly slice the avocado.

3. Mix the spinach, avocado and mallow flowers in a large bowl.

4. Prepare the vinaigrette by mixing the olive oil and balsamic vinegar. Add salt and pepper to taste.

5. Pour the vinaigrette over the salad, toss gently and serve chilled. Enjoy this salad, rich in flavor and health benefits!

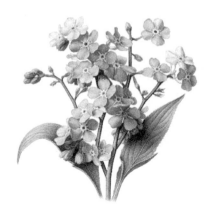

MYOSOTIS
(MYOSOTIS)

NATURE'S DISCREET ELOQUENCE

We're off to discover forget-me-nots, the little blue flower symbolizing remembrance and eternal love, with lesser-known properties just as interesting as its more famous peers.

Forget-me-nots, commonly known as "Myosotis", are a plant with strong symbolism, often linked to love and remembrance. These delicate flowers with their blue petals adorn gardens and wastelands in many parts of the world. Forget-me-nots are often associated with various myths and legends, evoking stories of lost love and eternal remembrance. But beyond its delicate appearance and rich symbolism, forget-me-not is also endowed with little-known medicinal properties. It has traditionally been used to treat respiratory and urinary disorders, and its infusion is renowned for its diuretic and expectorant properties. Although less well-known in phytotherapy than other plants, forget-me-nots offer a range of benefits that deserve greater recognition.

In the kitchen Forget-me-nots, with their **delicate, bluish hues, can** be used to **embellish dishes**. It is particularly used to **decorate and add a floral touch** to various dishes, such as salads and desserts. Forget-me-nots are appreciated not only for their charming appearance, but also for their **medicinal properties**. Young leaves can be eaten in salads, adding a **delicate, slightly spicy note** to the dish. As an infusion, forget-me-not is a **soothing drink**, promoting respiratory and digestive well-being. Its mildness makes it an ideal choice for those seeking to incorporate botanical elements into their diet without overpowering the flavors of the dish. Incorporating forget-me-nots into the kitchen pays tribute to its discreet beauty and wealth of beneficial compounds, while delicately awakening the taste buds. Be careful, however, to **select** it carefully **and consume it in moderation**, to enjoy its benefits and beauty in the kitchen in a healthy way.

HEALING WITH FORGET-ME-NOTS

- To **soothe the respiratory tract**, infuse a tablespoon of forget-me-not flowers in a cup of boiling water for 10 minutes. Strain and drink twice a day.

- **For urinary problems**, use forget-me-nots as a herbal tea, infusing the flowers in boiling water and drinking regularly.

- For **skin irritations**, prepare a poultice of crushed fresh forget-me-not flowers and apply to the affected area.

- If you have **a persistent cough,** an infusion of forget-me-not may be beneficial, thanks to its expectorant properties.

- To **improve memory and concentration,** regularly incorporate forget-me-nots into your diet, or drink its infusion regularly.

- For **sore throats,** gargle with a cooled infusion of forget-me-not several times a day.

- For **skin and acne** problems, apply a decoction of forget-me-nots directly to the skin as a natural tonic.

FORGET-ME-NOTS IN THE KITCHEN

Forget-Me-Not Summer Salad

INGREDIENTS: 100 g young forget-me-not leaves, 1 tomato, 1 cucumber, 50 g feta cheese, 1 tbsp olive oil, 1 tsp balsamic vinegar, salt, pepper.

- Wash and finely dice the tomatoes and cucumber.

- Crumble the feta cheese.

- Mix the vegetables, feta and young forget-me-not leaves in a bowl.

- In a bowl, prepare the vinaigrette with the olive oil, balsamic vinegar, salt and pepper.

- Drizzle vinaigrette over salad and toss gently.

- Serve chilled and enjoy your salad enriched by the delicate presence of forget-me-nots!

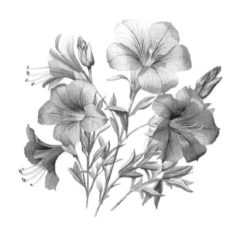

FIREWEED
(EPILOBIUM)

FOR EVERYDAY WELL-BEING

Let's discover fireweed, a medicinal plant renowned for its therapeutic properties, found in many temperate regions. It is best known for its benefits for the prostate and urinary system.

Fireweed, found mainly in temperate regions of the northern hemisphere, has been used for centuries for its medicinal virtues. In particular, it is recognized for its beneficial effects on the urinary system and prostate, as well as for its anti-inflammatory and antioxidant properties.

Native peoples in various regions used it to treat skin diseases, gastrointestinal disorders and urinary tract infections. Various species of fireweed were used in traditional medicine by the Greeks and Romans. These plants, with their generally pink or purple flowers, continue to attract the interest of herbalists and natural health practitioners.

In the kitchen

Fireweed can also find a place in our kitchens. The young leaves and shoots can be eaten raw or cooked, and are a **rich source of vitamins A and C**, while being **low in calories**. The leaves can be added to salads or cooked as a vegetable, while the slightly sweet flowers can be used to decorate dishes or make herbal teas. **An antioxidant**, fireweed is an excellent addition to meals for those seeking to combat free radicals. This medicinal plant also has **anti-inflammatory properties, making it a** wise choice for those suffering from chronic inflammatory conditions. Adding fireweed to our diet can help **promote prostate and urinary system health**, while **providing essential nutrients and beneficial phytochemicals**. Fireweed is also an excellent choice for those looking to add more wild plants to their diet, as it offers a variety of tastes and textures. Nevertheless, its culinary use is less widespread, but willowherb is gaining recognition as part of a balanced diet for its therapeutic and nutritional benefits.

TREATING YOURSELF WITH FIREWEED

- For **prostate problems**, prepare an infusion by adding a tablespoon of fireweed to a cup of boiling water. Leave to infuse for 10 minutes, then strain. Drink this infusion two or three times a day.

- For **urinary disorders**, drink fireweed tea regularly, adding a teaspoon of dried flowers to a cup of boiling water and leaving to infuse for around 10 minutes.

- For **skin inflammations**, apply a willowherb poultice to the affected area. Make a decoction of fresh plant and apply with a clean cloth.

- To relieve **digestive problems**, drink fireweed tea regularly. Add a teaspoon of dried herb to a cup of hot water, steep for 10 minutes, strain and drink.

- In case of **diarrhea,** take a teaspoon of dried fireweed leaves, infuse in boiling water for 10 minutes, and drink this preparation three times a day until improvement.

- For **mouth infections,** use fireweed as a mouthwash. Infuse a tablespoon of flowers in a cup of boiling water for 10 minutes, strain and use the lukewarm solution.

FIREWEED IN THE KITCHEN

Green Salad with Fireweed

INGREDIENTS: A few young fireweed leaves, 200 g salad greens (lettuce, arugula, etc.), 1 tomato, 1 cucumber, 1 tbsp olive oil, 1 tbsp balsamic vinegar, salt and pepper.

1. Wash and chop baby fireweed leaves, salad greens, tomatoes and cucumbers.

2. Mix all the vegetables in a bowl.

3. In a small bowl, combine the olive oil, balsamic vinegar, salt and pepper to create the vinaigrette.

4. Pour the dressing over the salad and toss well before serving. This salad is a great way to incorporate fireweed into your daily diet and enjoy its many health benefits. What's more, it's delicious!

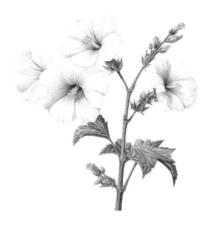

MARSHMALLOW
(ALTHAEA OFFICINALIS)

FOR SOFT SKIN AND A SOOTHED BODY

Let's stop off in Europe and discover a plant with unsuspected virtues and a rich history: the marshmallow, not the confectionery, but the plant from which it originates.

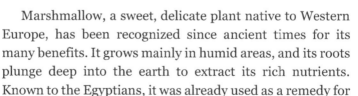

Marshmallow, a sweet, delicate plant native to Western Europe, has been recognized since ancient times for its many benefits. It grows mainly in humid areas, and its roots plunge deep into the earth to extract its rich nutrients. Known to the Egyptians, it was already used as a remedy for its soothing and softening properties. The Greeks and

Romans also appreciated it, notably for treating throat and stomach irritations. Over time, its use diversified, and it found its place in the European pharmacopoeia, both for its medicinal and dietary properties. Marshmallow's popularity peaked in the Middle Ages, when herbalists recommended it for everything from insect bites to stomach ulcers. The name "marshmallow" comes from the Latin "althaea", meaning "to heal". Its history is therefore deeply rooted in its ability to soothe and heal.

In the kitchen

Marshmallow isn't just a sweet confection enjoyed at campfires. In fact, its origins lie in the plant itself. The **mucilaginous roots** of the marshmallow plant were used to prepare a sweet to soothe the throat. Today, marshmallow is used in many recipes, from desserts to soups. Its tender, lightly scented leaves can be added to salads. As for the roots, they are **rich in mucilage**, a substance with **emollient and anti-inflammatory** properties. This makes them ideal for making throat-soothing syrups or decoctions. What's more, this plant is also a veritable treasure trove of health benefits. In addition to its soothing properties, it is also an **expectorant** and helps fight respiratory infections. In natural medicine, it is often prescribed for its gentle action on the digestive system, soothing inflammation and promoting healthy digestion. Its sweet fragrance and medicinal virtues make marshmallow a plant to be rediscovered in cooking and herbal medicine.

HEALING WITH MARSHMALLOW

- **Coughs and sore throats**: infuse a teaspoon of dried marshmallow root in a cup of hot water for 10 minutes. Strain and drink three times a day to soothe the throat.

- **Skin burns and irritations**: Apply a poultice of fresh marshmallow leaves directly to the affected area.

- **Constipation**: Take a teaspoon of marshmallow root powder and mix with a glass of water. Drink this before bedtime to promote smooth intestinal transit.

- **Urinary tract irritation**: drink a decoction made from one tablespoon of marshmallow root in 250 ml of water, three times a day.

- **Gastric ulcers**: mix a teaspoon of powdered marshmallow root in a glass of cold water, leave to stand for an hour, then drink.

- **Eczema**: Make a decoction of marshmallow root and use it as a lotion to soothe itching.

- **Sunburn**: Apply a paste made from crushed marshmallow leaves to soothe and moisturize the skin.

MARSHMALLOW IN THE KITCHEN

Creamy marshmallow soup

INGREDIENTS: 200 g marshmallow roots, 1 onion, 2 garlic cloves, 2 potatoes, 1 tbsp olive oil, 1 tsp salt, 1 l water, pepper to taste, crème fraîche (optional).

1. Peel and finely chop the onion and garlic. Peel the potatoes and cut into small cubes.

2. In a saucepan, heat the olive oil and sauté the onion and garlic until translucent.

3. Add the potato cubes, marshmallow roots, salt and water.

4. Bring to the boil, then reduce the heat and simmer until the potatoes are tender, about 20 minutes.

5. Blend the soup until smooth. Adjust seasoning with salt and pepper.

6. Serve hot, topped with crème fraîche if desired. Enjoy your meal!

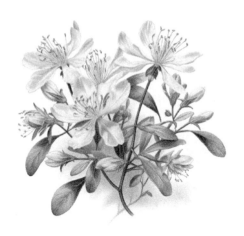

ST. JOHN'S WORT
(HYPERICUM PERFORATUM)

A NATURAL TREASURE FOR THE MOOD

Let's discover a thousand-year-old European plant which, in addition to its culinary uses, is best known for its mood-enhancing benefits: St. John's Wort.

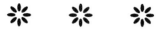

St. John's Wort, with its small, bright yellow flowers, is a plant native to Europe, but also spreading to Asia and North Africa. Its properties have been recognized since ancient times. The Greeks and Romans used it to treat a variety of ailments. In the Middle Ages, it was associated with religious beliefs and protection against evil spirits. The ancients believed that St John's Wort had the power to drive out demons. Over the centuries, St John's Wort became an essential medicinal herb, especially in Europe, where it was considered to have healing and soothing properties. More recently, in the 20th century, its antidepressant properties came to the fore, making this humble plant a natural remedy for melancholy and mild depression. Today, this luminous plant continues to light up our gardens, forests and, more discreetly, our medicinal preparations.

In the kitchen

St. John's Wort is less present in our kitchens than in our pharmacies, but it is not without culinary interest. Its leaves can be added to salads, adding a slightly bitter touch. St John's wort oil, obtained by macerating the flowers in olive oil, has **anti-inflammatory** properties and is used both in cooking and for external applications. Although not commonly used in gastronomy, it can be surprisingly effective as a secret ingredient in vinaigrettes or sauces to subtly spice up a dish. A natural **antiseptic**, oil can also be used to preserve other foods. But beware of overuse: some people may be sensitive to St. John's Wort and develop photosensitivity. Combining it with other herbs, such as thyme or rosemary, can not only balance its flavor, but also modulate its effects. It should therefore be used with discretion, in keeping with its medicinal use.

TREATMENT WITH ST JOHN'S WORT

- **Mild depression**: Infuse 1 to 2 teaspoons of dried St. John's Wort flowers in a cup of boiling water for 10 minutes. Drink this infusion once a day.

- **Burns and cuts**: Apply a St. John's wort-based ointment to the affected area to facilitate healing.

- **Muscle pain**: massage St. John's wort oil into sore areas to soothe pain.

- **Sleep disorders**: drink an infusion of St. John's Wort before bedtime to promote peaceful sleep.

- **Skin inflammations**: To relieve eczema and psoriasis, gently apply St. John's Wort oil to the affected areas.

- **Insect bites**: To soothe itching, dab the stung area with absorbent cotton soaked in St. John's Wort oil.

- If you have **bruises or contusions**: Applying St. John's wort oil can help reduce the appearance and pain of bruises.

ST JOHN'S WORT IN THE KITCHEN

Soothing herbal tea with St John's wort

INGREDIENTS: 1 tablespoon dried St. John's Wort flowers, 1 teaspoon honey, 1 slice lemon, 250 ml water.

1. Bring the water to the boil.
2. Place dried St John's Wort flowers in a cup.
3. Pour the boiling water over the flowers.

4. Leave to infuse for 5 to 10 minutes.

5. Strain and add honey and lemon slice to taste. Drink warm and enjoy this soothing drink!

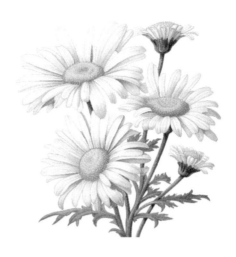

OXEYE DAISY
(LEUCANTHEMUM VULGARE)

THE BRILLIANCE OF THE EUROPEAN GARDEN

Let's dive into the meadows of Europe to discover an emblematic flower: the Oxeye daisy, star of the fields, which has charmed poets and inspired many legends.

The Oxeye daisy, with its radiant white petals and bright yellow heart, is one of Europe's most recognized flowers. It has stood proudly in meadows, fields and forest edges for centuries. This simple yet powerful flower has witnessed many historic events, blending with poetry, folk medicine and belief. In ancient Greece, the daisy was thought to be the flower of the goddess Artemis, protector of women and fertility. During the Middle Ages in Europe, it was often used in rites and love potions. Its popularity has endured through the ages, where it has been celebrated by poets, artists and even used in rituals to divine love - "he loves me, a little, a lot...". With its deep roots in folklore and tradition, the Great Daisy remains an emblematic flower of natural beauty and simplicity.

In the kitchen

The Oxeye daisyis not only a pleasure for the eyes, it also has a place on our plates. Its young, slightly bitter leaves can be added to salads to give them a **unique flavor**. The flower petals, meanwhile, offer a delicate taste and can be sprinkled on desserts or used to make refreshing drinks. Rich in **antioxidants** and **vitamin C,** these flowers also offer numerous health benefits. In traditional medicine, daisies have been used as a **remedy for coughs**, sore throats and various inflammations. Infusing the flowers can help **soothe the digestive and nervous systems**. If you're looking for a unique floral touch to your dishes, or a delicious drink to help you relax, think Oxeye daisy. But always in moderation, because like all plants, it's important to know the appropriate quantities to consume.

HEALING WITH THE OXEYE DAISY

- **For skin irritations**, prepare an infusion of daisy flowers. Use this infusion to gently cleanse irritated skin.

- To **soothe tired eyes**, infuse a few petals in hot water. Leave to cool, then soak two compresses in the infusion and place them on your eyelids for a few minutes.

- **For sore throats**, make an herbal tea with daisy flowers. Drink 2 to 3 times a day.

- To **reduce inflammation,** crush daisy flowers to extract the juice. Apply directly to the inflamed area.

- **For rheumatism**, prepare a poultice with fresh flowers. Apply to painful areas.

- For **rashes** or acne, an infusion of daisy flowers applied topically can help soothe and purify the skin.

- **To boost the immune system**, drink daisy flower tea regularly.

OXEYE DAISY IN THE KITCHEN

Fresh salad with oxeye daisy

INGREDIENTS: 100 g baby spinach, 1 handful oxeye daisy, 50 g feta cheese, 10 cherry tomatoes, 1 tbsp olive oil, 1 tsp balsamic vinegar, salt and pepper.

1. Wash the spinach shoots and daisy flowers.

2. Cut the feta cheese into small cubes.

3. In a salad bowl, combine the spinach, feta cheese, halved cherry tomatoes and daisy flowers.

4. In a separate bowl, prepare the vinaigrette by mixing the olive oil, balsamic vinegar, salt and pepper.

5. Pour the vinaigrette over the salad, toss well and serve chilled. Enjoy your meal!

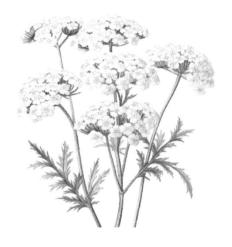

YARROW
(ACHILLEA MILLEFOLIUM)

FOR NATURAL HEALING

Discover yarrow, a medicinal plant used for centuries for its health benefits, and a veritable treasure of the European countryside.

Yarrow is a plant that has found its place in the history of phytotherapy. It takes its name from the Greek hero Achilles, who, according to mythology, used this plant to heal his soldiers' wounds during the Trojan War. This plant with its small white or pink flowers, frequently found in the fields and meadows of Europe and Asia, has been used throughout history for its medicinal properties. It was a key element in European folklore and was often used in magical rituals to ward off evil. Moreover, its virtues have been hailed in the pharmacopoeias of many civilizations, from the ancient Egyptians to the Romans, via traditional healers in China. It is also very much in evidence in traditional European medicine, where it was used in particular to aid digestion and treat female diseases.

In the kitchen

Yarrow, despite its powerful medicinal properties, has also found its way into our kitchens. Its delicately scented leaves can be incorporated into salads, offering a **bitter flavor** that can balance out rich dishes. The tender young leaves can be eaten raw, while the more mature ones are usually cooked to reduce their bitterness. The flowers, meanwhile, are often used to infuse herbal teas, renowned for their **digestive benefits**. As well as improving digestion, yarrow is **anti-inflammatory**, helping to soothe upset stomachs. It also has **diuretic properties** that can help eliminate excess fluids from the body. If you're looking for a natural ingredient to enhance your dishes while enjoying its many health benefits, yarrow is certainly an option to explore. However, as with all medicinal herbs, consumption in moderation is recommended.

TREATING YOURSELF WITH YARROW

- **For painful periods**: Infuse 1 teaspoon of dried yarrow flowers in a cup of boiling water for 10 minutes. Strain and drink twice a day.

- **For digestive disorders**, prepare a decoction with a tablespoon of dried plant in a cup of water. Bring to the boil and leave to infuse for 10 minutes. Drink lukewarm before meals.

- **For nosebleeds,** infuse a few yarrow flowers in boiling water for 10 minutes. Leave to cool, soak a compress and apply to the nose.

- **For cuts and small wounds**, apply a paste of crushed yarrow leaves directly to the wound. It has healing properties.

- **To relieve skin inflammation**, prepare a concentrated infusion and use it as a lotion on affected areas.

- **For headaches,** place a sachet of dried flowers under your pillow to benefit from the soothing effects of yarrow.

YARROW IN THE KITCHEN

Relaxing herbal tea with yarrow

INGREDIENTS: 2 teaspoons yarrow flowers, 1 teaspoon peppermint, 1 teaspoon chamomile, 250 ml boiling water, honey (optional).

1. Mix yarrow flowers, peppermint and chamomile in a container.
2. Pour the boiling water over the mixed herbs.
3. Cover and leave to infuse for 10 minutes.

4. Strain the infusion to remove the herbs.

5. If you like, add a little honey for sweetness. Enjoy warm and feel the relaxation after a long day.

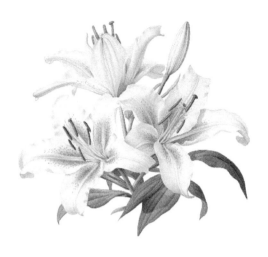

LILY
(LILIUM)

The symbol of purity and majesty

A symbol of royalty and purity throughout the ages, the lily is much more than just an ornamental flower. Its rich history and varied uses still fascinate us today.

The lily, with its majestic beauty and long, sturdy stems, is a flower that has captivated people since ancient times. Associated with Greek and Roman mythology, the lily was a symbol of the goddess Hera and is often depicted in various legends and stories. With its regal allure, it's not surprising that the lily was adopted by the kings of France as their emblem. This symbol has been taken up through the ages and has become the sign of royalty and purity, particularly in connection with the Virgin Mary in Christianity. From ancient Egypt to the European Renaissance, the lily has been represented in art, sculpture and literature, testifying to its predominant place in world culture. Its delicate petals, which can vary from pure white to deep red or golden yellow, are often associated with restoration and rebirth.

In the kitchen

The lily, often seen as an ornamental flower, has unsuspected culinary properties. Its buds and petals are **edible** and have been used in various cuisines, particularly in Asia. Rich in antioxidants, they offer not only a decorative touch, but also a nutritional contribution. In China, lily buds, known as "Bai He", are traditionally used in soups for their ability to **moisturize** the skin and **soothe** coughs. The root, or bulb, of the lily is also eaten in some regions, providing a crunchy texture and mild taste, similar to potatoes or turnips. **Rich in vitamin C and fiber,** the bulb can be steamed, fried or boiled. But before using them in cooking, it's essential to check that the lily you've chosen is edible, as not all varieties are. What's more, this beautiful flower is also used to create health-giving infusions. So the next time you admire a lily, remember that it's not just a beautiful flower, but also a culinary treasure.

HEALING WITH LILIES

- **For light burns**, crush a few fresh lily petals to make a gel. Apply the gel directly to the burn to soothe the pain.

- **For sunburn,** prepare an infusion of lily petals. Leave to cool, then use as a compress on the affected areas to soothe the skin.

- For **dry skin problems**, use lily oil. This oil, extracted from the bulbs, is renowned for its moisturizing properties.

- **For freckles**, apply petal gel directly to the spots to help reduce them over time.

- If you have **skin irritations,** use lily petal gel as a soothing balm.

- **For insomnia,** make a tea with a few lily petals. Drink it before going to bed for a peaceful night's sleep.

- For **respiratory problems**, inhale the aroma of lily flowers to help you breathe more easily and soothe your respiratory system.

LILY IN THE KITCHEN

Lily petal salad

INGREDIENTS: Well-washed lily petals (edible varieties), 50 g arugula, 1/2 sliced cucumber, 10 halved cherry tomatoes, vinaigrette of your choice, 1 tsp toasted sesame seeds.

1. Start by gently combining the lily petals, arugula, cucumber and cherry tomatoes in a large bowl.

2. Drizzle the salad with your favorite vinaigrette.
3. Sprinkle with toasted sesame seeds.
4. Serve chilled and enjoy this fragrant and original salad!

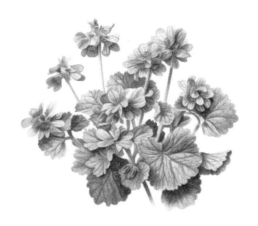

GROUND IVY
(GLECHOMA HEDERACEA)

FOR FREE BREATHING

Although often overshadowed by its climbing counterpart, ground ivy is a treasure trove of benefits that we're about to discover. Let's embark on a journey through its history and uses.

This small ground cover plant, commonly found in the undergrowth and meadows of Europe, has been used for centuries as a medicinal plant. Contrary to what its name might suggest, it bears no relation to the climbing ivy with which we are all familiar. Ground ivy is a perennial plant with small, heart-shaped leaves and tiny purple flowers that bloom in spring. In the Middle Ages, it was commonly used to treat tuberculosis and other respiratory ailments thanks to its expectorant properties. It was also used as a remedy for snakebites and was considered to protect against the evil eye. Over time, its use diversified and it became a prized plant in various cultures. Monks, for example, used ground ivy to make certain beers before hops became the norm.

In the kitchen

Although less famous than other herbs, **ground ivy** has a delicate mint-like fragrance, making it an excellent addition to a variety of dishes. Its leaves can be chopped and added to salads to give them a **fresh flavor**. They have also been used to flavor traditional beers. Beyond its culinary uses, Ground Ivy is **rich in vitamins** and **antioxidants**. Its **expectorant** properties make it beneficial for those suffering from congestion or respiratory ailments. In infusion, it can help **clear the respiratory tract** and relieve sore throats. However, in large quantities, it can have narcotic effects, so it is essential to use it in moderation. What's more, like all herbs, it's important to be sure of its provenance, and that it hasn't been treated with pesticides or other chemicals.

HEALING WITH GROUND IVY

- **For coughs**: infuse a teaspoon of dried leaves in a cup of boiling water for 10 minutes. Drink this infusion 2 or 3 times a day to soothe coughs.

- **For sore throats**: crush a few fresh ivy leaves and mix with a teaspoon of honey. Take this mixture 2 times a day.

- **For insomnia:** add a teaspoon of Ground Ivy to a cup of hot water. Leave to infuse for 10 minutes and drink before going to bed.

- **For insect bites:** crush a few fresh leaves to extract the juice and apply directly to the bite to relieve itching.

- **For cuts and scrapes**: crush the leaves into a paste and apply to the affected area. This can help disinfect and heal the wound more quickly.

- **Respiratory problems**: inhale the aroma of a warm infusion of Ground Ivy to help clear the respiratory tract.

GROUND IVY IN THE KITCHEN

Ground Ivy Salad

INGREDIENTS: 200 g young ground ivy shoots, 50 g walnuts, 50 g feta cheese, 1 tbsp cider vinegar, 2 tbsp olive oil, 1 tsp mustard, salt, pepper.

1. Wash and squeeze out the young shoots of ground ivy.

2. In a large bowl, combine the sprouts, walnuts and crumbled feta cheese.

3. In a small bowl, prepare the vinaigrette by mixing vinegar, mustard, olive oil, salt and pepper.

4. Pour the vinaigrette over the salad, toss well and serve chilled. Enjoy your meal!

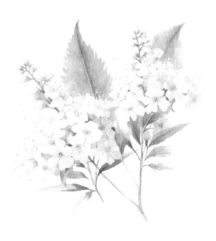

MEADOWSWEET
(FILIPENDULA ULMARIA)

FOR PEACE OF MIND

Now let's discover a European plant that evokes flowery meadows and gentle rivers: Reine-des-Prés, a gem of phytotherapy.

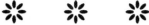

Nicknamed for its majestic stature and graceful white flowers, meadowsweet evokes the beauty of European meadows. Since ancient times, this plant has been recognized for its medicinal virtues. The Celts, then the Romans, used Meadowsweet as a sacred plant and to treat various ailments. Over time, it became one of the most widely used plants in traditional pharmacopoeia. Its fame peaked in the 19th century, when scientists isolated from its flowers a substance with analgesic and anti-inflammatory properties, which was to form the basis of aspirin. Reine-des-Prés is thus intimately linked to the history of modern medicine. Its delicate flowers give off a sweet almond fragrance, reminiscent of warm summer days.

In the kitchen

Reine-des-Prés has a sweet, aromatic flavor slightly reminiscent of almond and vanilla. It can enhance your beverages, especially infusions and syrups. Used in Europe for centuries, it goes perfectly with fruit salads or desserts, adding a sweet, floral touch. **Rich in flavonoids** and **salicylic acid**, it has **anti-inflammatory** and **analgesic properties, making it** an excellent option for soothing aches and pains. In addition to its delicate flavor, its diuretic properties make it an excellent choice for detoxifying infusions. It also adds a slight sweetness to liqueurs and cocktails. However, it is essential to dose it with care, as its taste can quickly become overpowering. In modern gastronomy, chefs exploit its subtle flavours in sweet and savoury creations, bringing out its unique character. But beware: it's important not to consume large quantities, as Reine-des-Prés, like aspirin, can cause gastric irritation in large doses.

HEALING WITH MEADOWSWEET

- **For joint pain**, prepare an infusion by putting a teaspoon of dried flowers in a cup of boiling water. Leave to infuse for 10 minutes, then strain. Drink 2 to 3 cups a day.

- **To soothe headaches**, take a handful of Meadowsweet flowers and boil them in half a liter of water for 5 minutes. Leave to infuse for 10 minutes, strain and drink.

- **If you suffer from indigestion**, mix a teaspoon of dried flowers in a cup of boiling water. Leave to infuse for 10 minutes, strain and drink after each meal.

- **For menstrual pain,** take an infusion of Meadowsweet two or three times a day, starting a few days before your period begins.

- **For water retention problems**, prepare an infusion with a teaspoon of flowers and drink 2 to 3 cups a day.

- **In the event of fever,** Meadowsweet's sudorific action helps bring the temperature down. Drink 3 cups of infusion a day until symptoms improve.

MEADOWSWEET IN THE KITCHEN

Soothing herbal tea with Reine-des-Prés

INGREDIENTS: 2 tablespoons dried Meadowsweet flowers, 1 tablespoon honey, zest of half a lemon, 500 ml water.

1. Bring the water to the boil.

2. Place the dried flowers and lemon zest in a teapot.

3. Pour the boiling water into the teapot and leave to infuse for 10 minutes.

4. Strain the mixture to remove the flowers and zest.

5. Add the honey and mix well.

6. Serve hot and enjoy this relaxing, fragrant herbal tea!

CONCLUSION

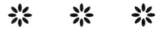

Final thoughts on Edible Flowers

As we close the pages of this botanical journey, one thing is clear: edible flowers are much more than a mere ornament or ephemeral decoration on our dishes. They embody a symphony of colors, flavors, textures and health benefits, offering a world of unexplored possibilities for gourmets, the curious and those seeking to reconnect with nature.

Travelling the globe, from Mediterranean Europe to tropical forests to the vast wilds of North America, we've come to appreciate the richness and diversity of edible flowers. Each one tells a story, whether linked to ancient culinary traditions, medicinal rituals or simply the sheer beauty of nature.

It's amazing how, despite the modernity and technology that surround us, simple flowers can still fill us with wonder. They remind us of the importance of simplicity, of taking time to savor the present moments and finding pleasure in the little things. In an age when speed is often of the essence, edible flowers invite us to slow down, pay attention and cherish our environment.

One of the most valuable lessons we can learn from this book is the notion of respect. Respect for nature, which offers us these treasures, but also for the cultures and traditions that have preserved and passed on the knowledge of edible flowers through the generations. In our quest for novelty, it's essential to remember that each flower has its own balance in the ecosystem, and that our desire to consume them must be balanced by a responsible and sustainable approach.

This book also aims to stimulate creativity. Each flower described here is an invitation to experiment in the kitchen, creating new dishes, refreshing drinks or natural remedies. The possibilities are endless and, with a little imagination, edible flowers can become the stars of your table.

But beyond the kitchen, there's a deeper dimension to explore. Integrating flowers into our diet is a way of reconnecting with the Earth, acknowledging our dependence on her and celebrating her generosity. It's a way of reminding ourselves that we are an integral part of a whole, interconnected with nature and other living beings.

Before concluding, it's important to stress that, although this book is an introduction to edible flowers, it's crucial to continue your research, consult experts and always exercise caution. Not all the world's flowers are edible, and some may even be toxic. Responsible consumption is therefore essential.

Finally, I hope you find this book a source of inspiration, whether to add a floral touch to your meals, deepen your knowledge of botany or simply take a moment to appreciate the beauty that surrounds us. May every flower you encounter from now on be a reminder of the magic of nature and the richness of our cultural and gastronomic heritage.

Thank you for accompanying me on this exploration of the world's edible flowers. May this book awaken in you a renewed curiosity and deep appreciation for the treasures nature has to offer.

Thanks

I would like to express my gratitude to all those who have made this book possible. To the many researchers and authors who have preserved and interpreted this art of consuming edible flowers. To the editorial team who carefully crafted every page of this book. And above all, to you, dear readers, for your interest.

Give your honest opinion on Amazon!

Your suggestions and criticisms are invaluable.

They make every reading experience even more satisfying!

Thank you very much for reading my book.

I wish you all the success you deserve!

Source Images

The author and publisher would particularly like to thank the following websites:

www.pxhere.com/

www.freepik.com

Printed in France by Amazon
Brétigny-sur-Orge, FR